REVISION NOTES

FOR

SENIOR NURSES

☐ ☐ Medicine ②

John F Morris, SRN RNT

Senior Tutor, Portsmouth Group School of Nursing
Examiner to the General Nursing Council of England and Wales

John C Small, SRN RMN RNT

Senior Tutor, Portsmouth Group School of Nursing
Examiner to the General Nursing Council of England and Wales

WILLIAM HEINEMANN MEDICAL BOOKS LTD

LONDON

First published 1978
© J F Morris and J C Small 1978
ISBN 0 433 30432 4
Typeset by H Charlesworth & Co Ltd, Huddersfield
and printed by Redwood Burn Ltd., Trowbridge and Esher

CONTENTS

Josie Finucane.
Marian T. Bose

PREFACE

This companion volume to Revision Notes for Senior Nurses:
Vol.1 is directed to all grades of nurses who wish to revise the
salient points of some common medical conditions, and together
with the first volume completes the medical series, Read in conjunction with the previously published edition on Surgery, the
volumes will be of interest to all nurses who are studying on a
systematic basis during revisionary and other study periods.

   The format of previous books has been welcomed by nurses
in different stages of their training and we have therefore retained
the style of presentation.

   Our thanks are due to all who have aided us in the preparation
of this series and in particular to our students past and present
whose searching questions have been of great value.

JFM
JCS

Mouth and salivary glands

Oesophagus

Stomach

Duodenum

Small &
large
intestine

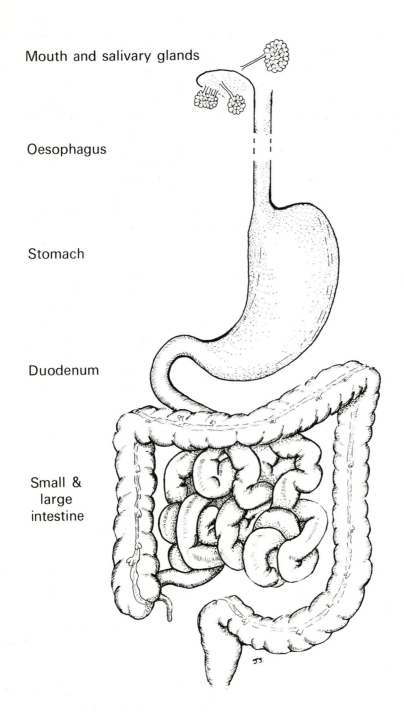

1 Common signs and symptoms of gastro-intestinal disorders

It may be of benefit if, before discussing gastro-intestinal disorders, a brief outline of the relevant anatomy and physiology is presented.

The alimentary tract consists of the mouth, pharynx, oesophagus, stomach and intestines. The process of digestion involves both mechanical and chemical factors, the mechanical being mastication and swallowing, plus the movements of the intestines, the chemical processes resulting from the constituents of saliva (ptyaline etc), the gastro-intestinal juices and other secretions. Any alteration in the mechanical, or change in the chemical processes can adversely affect the individual e.g. food which has been inadequately masticated will lead to indigestion, absence of movement in the small intestine (ileus) is of serious consequence, sluggishness of the large bowel from whatever cause leads to constipation.

The necessity of continual oral toilet, especially in the very ill, dehydrated patient is well known, the dry mouth present due to the poor supply of saliva and its constituents. The cleansing and moistening effect of saliva is absent, resulting if neglected, in parotitis. Conversely peptic ulceration may be due to too much hydrochloric acid in the stomach. Oesophagitis may be due to a reflux of gastric contents into the cardiac end of the oesophagus. Thus, absence of, or over secretion of normal enzymes can have an ill effect. Similarly, diminished or lack of intestinal movement will also have adverse effects.

Basically the alimentary tract is a long tube with common features along its length. It consists, but for a very short section of the oesophagus, of involuntary muscle with a lining of mucous membrane.

Modifications exist along the tract to cater for somewhat differing functions. Such modifications would be the stomach, the most widely dilated portion, with the muscle layers possessing an extra oblique layer. The presence of the numerous villi of the small intestine allow for maximum absorption, the ability of the large intestine to absorb water and salts and so make the faecal contents more solid. Other relevant details with particular application to diseased conditions will be discussed under the appropriate headings.

The main symptoms of gastro-intestinal disease are pain, vomiting, nausea, flatulence, heartburn, waterbrash and chronic diarrhoea.

Pain
Pain is probably the most common symptom complained of by patients with gastro-intestinal disease. The site of the pain

PAIN

VOMITING

NAUSEA

FLATULENCE

HEARTBURN

WATERBRASH

CHRONIC DIARRHOEA

experienced in gastric ulceration is usually localised in the epigastrium. The timing of the pain is also of significance in assisting the physician in his diagnosis. With gastric ulcers the pain is experienced about an hour after a meal, but the timing is often irregular. Duodenal ulcers cause pain to develop several hours after a meal when the stomach is empty and is often referred to as hunger pain.

Colic is a form of pain arising from the spasm of any hollow muscular organ and tends to be spasmodic in character. The pain in intestinal colic usually comes and goes in a succession of waves rising to a peak and then subsiding. This type of pain would occur for example in acute intestinal obstruction.

Inflammation of the peritoneum causes pain which is severe, sharp and usually localised over the area of inflammation, an example being the steady pain experienced in the later stages of acute appendicitis.

Nausea and vomiting
There are many causes of vomiting other than gastro-intestinal disorders. When the cause is of gastro-intestinal origin the vomiting is usually preceded by nausea. Conditions such as pyloric stenosis, intestinal obstruction, peritonitis, appendicitis and cholecystitis are examples which cause vomiting from diseased states.

The projectile nature and the quantity of material vomited in pyloric stenosis are well recognised by nurses. Similarly the faecal character of the vomitus in intestinal obstruction is also diagno-stic. Patients sometimes state that vomiting has given them a degree of relief from discomfort, which can occur in pyloric stenosis and this sign in itself may be indicative of some form of obstruction. Nurses should observe the type and character of any vomitus from whatever cause and report accordingly.

Flatulence
Flatulence may be considered as air or gas in the stomach, small intestine and large intestine.

Most people swallow some air with their meals but any unpleasant gas from the stomach can be an indication of achlor-hydria or pyloric obstruction. In intestinal obstruction the presence of gas in the gut causes distension and can be detected on X ray.

Heartburn and waterbrash
The above symptoms are unpleasant but not very significant to the nurse but waterbrash in which the mouth fills with saliva can be an indication of duodenal ulcer.

Diarrhoea
Diarrhoea is a significant symptom in such conditions as Crohn's disease and in diseases such as ulcerative colitis, diverticulitis, carcinoma of the colon and in the malabsorption syndromes.

Achalasia of the cardia

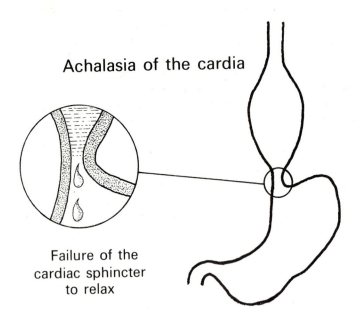

Failure of the
cardiac sphincter
to relax

Oesophagitis

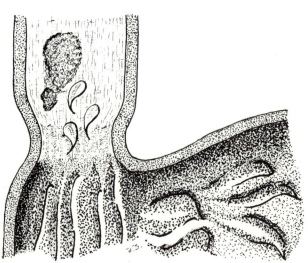

Reflux of gastric
contents
irritating
the oesophagus

2 The oesophagus

Achalasia of the Cardia

The chief symptoms complained of by the patient are dysphagia and regurgitation. It appears that the condition is due to some disorder of the motor function of the oesophagus in which there is absence of peristalsis in the lower two thirds of the structure resulting in failure of the cardiac sphincter to relax. The onset of the dysphagia is usually gradual with patients increasingly complaining of difficulty in swallowing. As the condition progresses a build up of food in the oesophagus occurs and the patient experiences some discomfort behind the sternum. In severe cases a spill over into the lungs results causing the patient to suffer recurrent attacks of pneumonia from the infected material entering the lungs.

Diagnosis is confirmed by radiological examination which shows the delay at the cardia, or in more severe cases a grossly distended oesophagus filled with the residue of food. Oesophagoscopy is performed in order to exclude some obstructive lesion. The nurse may be asked to carefully wash out the oesophagus prior to this procedure.

Treatment

The passage of a bougie is considered, this procedure forcibly ruptures the muscle fibres at the cardia and may in itself cause a cure. Drugs which will relax the sphincter are sometimes employed but this form of treatment is only effective for a very short period. The operative treatment is Heller's operation (cardiomyotomy) which often gives satisfactory results.

Oesophagitis

Any reflux of the acid gastric juice over a period of time will eventually affect the squamous epithelium which lines the oesophagus. The lining becomes inflamed and eroded and gives rise to pain which is felt under the sternum, or to frequent small bleeds which tend to cause anaemia in the patient.

Oesophagitis can occur in patients who suffer from hiatus hernia. The patient will complain of pain when lying flat or on stooping after a meal. It will be noted that such positions encourage the reflux of gastric material, the acidity of which irritates the mucous membrane of the oesophagus and so causing the symptoms. Diagnosis is by way of a barium meal and in order to demonstrate the reflux the patient is placed in the Trendelenburg position at the investigation.

Treatment is usually medical in which the patient is given alkaline preparations, advised to eat small frequent meals, and to sit well propped up in bed. Patients in hospital would probably have the head of the bed raised on blocks. Some patients however have to undergo surgery in which the hiatus hernia is repaired.

The structure
of the
stomach
contains

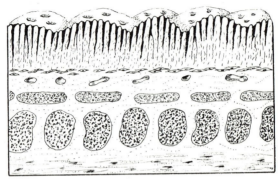

Mucous membrane
Submucous layer
Muscular layer
Peritoneum

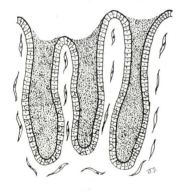

The mucous membrane
contains secretory
cells forming

Pepsin

Hydrochloric acid

Mucus

The intrinsic factor

3 The stomach and duodenum

Peptic ulceration
The stomach, as previously mentioned, is the most dilated
portion of the alimentary tract and its primary function is to act
as a reservoir for food. The peristaltic action of the stomach
walls, together with the action of the gastric secretions, mixes the
contents and prepares it for entry into the duodenum in a semi-
liquid state. The gastric juices contain some important constituents such as pepsin, hydrochloric acid, mucus and the intrinsic
factor of Castle, the latter being essential for normal haemopoiesis.
The juices are produced by specific cells situated in the stomach,
the control of their production being under both nervous and
hormonal mechanisms. The secretion of hydrochloric acid is
brought about by action of the vagus nerve. Acid can also be
secreted by the presence of food in the stomach whereby a
hormone-gastria is released from the antrum of the stomach.
The appetite stimulatory effect of the sight and smell of food
is well known. Most nurses are aware that the use of histamine
in certain gastric analysis tests is a powerful stimulant to the
secretion of hydrochloric acid.

Investigation of gastric disorders
When examing a patient with suspected gastric trouble the
physician will probably arrive at his diagnosis by using one or
more of the following methods.

1 Physical examination
The patient may be able to point with one finger to the area
in the epigastrium where he experiences pain. This is called
'pointing sign' and may suggest the presence of peptic ulceration.
 Palpation of the epigastrium when peptic ulceration is present
makes the patient give some visible evidence of pain i.e. there is
evidence of epigastric tenderness. In pyloric stenosis the examining physician is able to detect in many patients visible peristalsis.

2 X ray examination
A barium meal examination will give valuable information
regarding the presence of ulceration, rate of emptying and also
give information about the peristaltic action of the stomach.
Additionally it will also indicate any filling defects diaphrag-
matic herniation and evidence of carcinoma when present.

3 Gastroscopy
The gastroscope enables the examining physician to inspect the
interior of the stomach and in conjunction with other methods
confirm a diagnosis. *Biopsies* of the mucosa will also assist in
diagnosis.

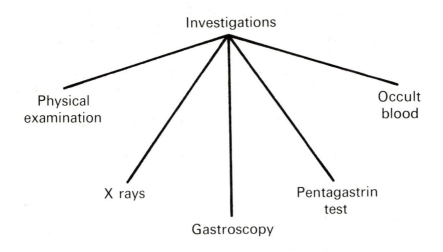

Investigations

Physical examination

X rays

Gastroscopy

Pentagastrin test

Occult blood

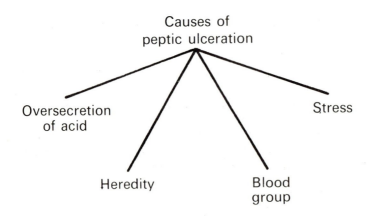

Causes of peptic ulceration

Oversecretion of acid

Heredity

Blood group

Stress

9

4 Pentagastrin test

The previously mentioned investigations are the particular province of the physician but nurse involvement is necessary in tests which measure the acid secretory capacity of the stomach.
The nursing duties for the above test involve:-

a Weighing the patient.

b Passing the naso gastric tube of the radio opaque type.

c Checking that a sufficiency of Pentagastrin (Peptavlon) is available. The usual amount required is six micrograms per kilogram of body weight.

d Ensuring that the suction pump is in working order.

e Ensuring that the supply of special flasks has been obtained, usually from the pharmacy.

f Correct labelling plus the exact recording of timing of the samples obtained.

g Making sure that the patient is aware of the forthcoming test.

5 Occult blood

The nurse will be required to obtain three to five consecutive stool specimens. The test will show a positive result in patients with active bleeding ulcers.

Aetiology of peptic ulcers

The term peptic ulcer usually refers to ulceration occurring in the stomach and the duodenum. It can also refer to ulcers found in the lower end of the oesophagus or to the anastomotic variety when the small intestine has been anastomosed to the stomach.

The cause of peptic ulceration is unknown but certain factors appear to predispose to the condition.

1 Oversecretion of hydrochloric acid.

2 Heredity, there is often a strong family history of peptic ulcers.

3 It has been established that people with blood group O are more likely to be affected.

4 Stress. People who have somewhat stressful occupations and who also tend to have hurried meals may also be likely to suffer from this condition.

Pathology

Peptic ulcers can be acute or chronic and may arise in the stomach, duodenum or occasionally in the lower end of the oesophagus. Acute ulcers may be present in an individual but not give rise to any symptoms and may not be diagnosed unless they cause complications such as haematemesis or perforation. They tend to heal fairly rapidly but can recur and may give notice of their presence by one or other of the above complications.

Clinical features
of
peptic ulceration

DYSPEPSIA

Intermittent & later
for longer periods.

PAIN

In the epigastrium, may
be relieved by food

VOMITING

May bring relief, if persistent
causes loss of weight

Clinical features

Although peptic ulceration may indicate its presence in many ways certain signs and symptoms are of significance.

Dyspepsia

In the early stages dyspepsia is notably intermittent in nature but later the patient experiences discomfort for much longer periods as the interval between attacks lessens.

Pain

Often pain is the major symptom complained of by the patient. The pain is usually felt in the epigastrium and the sufferer will point accurately to the centre of the epigastrium, which as already indicated, the physicians term the 'pointing sign'.

A characteristic feature of pain in peptic ulceration is its relationship to the presence or absence of food in the stomach. With duodenal ulceration the pain is similar to that of hunger and is consequently experienced when the stomach is empty. The partaking of a glass of milk with a biscuit will often give relief. It is this type of pain which wakes the patient at night, some patients will have the necessary relief to hand at the bedside.

Patients with gastric ulcers will complain that the pain occurs very shortly after a meal, usually about half to one hour after. These patients tend to eat very lightly because they know the taking of a meal will cause a degree of physical discomfort. Patients will also relate that they often have periods when they are completely free from pain, sometimes for many months.

Vomiting

Vomiting by the sufferer will often bring with it a feeling of relief. When the ulceration over a period of time has in turn brought about pyloric stenosis the patient will vomit material which has been in the stomach for some time, the stenosis being one obvious cause of delayed emptying. Persistent vomiting can result in some loss of weight.

Diagnosis

The diagnosis of peptic ulceration is usually confirmed by the investigations undertaken i.e. barium meal, gastroscopy and possibly gastric secretion tests and tests for occult blood.

Treatment

Rest

Perhaps rest is the most beneficial single factor in the treatment of peptic ulceration. Although it can be achieved at home, in many ways it is probably of more benefit if the patient is admitted to hospital, and except for toilet purposes, be confined to bed. It may also be easier for the patient to give up smoking

TREATMENT

Rest in bed

Stop smoking

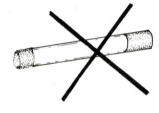

Eat non-irritating
food

Eat small meals
regularly

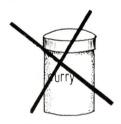

DRUGS

Antacids

Vagal paralysants

Liquorice preparations

when in hospital and under supervision. Smoking is considered by some authorities to delay healing and the nurse should therefore try to get the patient to give it up even if only for a few weeks.

Diet
Usually the patient is given frequent non-irritating meals in which milk would be the basis. A diet of two hourly milk feeds is often ordered, supplemented by such food items as junkets, custards and pureed dishes. Gradually as the symptoms disappear the patient is given a more normal diet, but obviously avoiding any highly spiced dishes and any food items which experience tells him he should avoid.

Drugs
Antacids such as magnesium hydroxide, calcium carbonate, bismuth carbonate, magnesium trisilicate and aluminium hydroxide are usually prescribed when the patient is admitted. At home many sufferers will take sodium bicarbonate but as the drug is readily absorbed it can, when taken over long periods, cause alkalosis. Antacids will neutralise the gastric acidity and if the pain is severe the physician will order the drug to be given frequently. Preparations such as Nulacin can be taken in tablet form, the patient chewing or sucking one whenever he feels epigastric pain.

Side effects of antacid therapy can be either diarrhoea or constipation. The nurse will report to the doctor these effects in order that a more balanced mixture may be ordered and so avoid the complications.

Other drugs used include drugs which will act as vagal paralysants, tranquillisers and drugs which are derivatives of liquorice, a preparation which appears to expedite the healing of ulcers.

An example of the former would be Propanthelin. The drug inhibits vagal stimulation thus decreasing the motility and secretory powers of the stomach. There are however certain unpleasant side effects such as a dry mouth or perhaps blurred vision or even urinary retention. The preparation is often ordered for patients who experience nocturnal pain and are thus awakened at night time.

Examples of the liquorice preparations would be Carbenoxolone (Biogastrone) or Caved S. These are frequently ordered when patients are hospitalised as in some patients certain degree of control is necessary. Side effects such as the retention of sodium and water or the lowering of potassium levels have been reported.

More recently drugs have been introduced which, following extensive clinical trials, appear to have given excellent clinical results. The preparations are
  1 Tagamet (Cimetidine)
  2 De-Nol.

Surgery is indicated
if

ULCERS
FAIL TO
HEAL

PYLORIC
STENOSIS
OCCURS

PERFORATION

SEVERE
HAEMATEMESIS

POSSIBLE
MALIGNANCY

15

Tagamet

The preparation is used for peptic ulcers and associated gastro-intestinal disorders such as reflux oesophagitis, and conditions whereby a reduction of gastric acid secretion would be of benefit. Briefly, the drug acts by blocking the secretion of histamine which is a potent stimulant of gastric acid.

The drug can be administered orally in either tablet form or as a flavoured syrup. It can also be given by injection.
The preparation is presented as follows

Tablets   200mgms.
Syrup   200mgms in 5mls.
Ampoules   200mgms in 2ml ampoules.

The oral dose is 200mgms three times daily, to be taken with meals plus one dose of 400mgms at bedtime. If necessary the dose may be increased to 400mgms at mealtimes together with the 400mgms at bedtime. The physician will monitor responses and alter the dose accordingly, but will probably also order the more familiar antacids to be given in conjunction with Tagamet until symptomatic relief is obtained.

Should there be any difficulty in administering the drug orally, i.e. vomiting or an unconscious patient, then the intravenous route can be used.

Side effects

Occasionally patients have developed mild but transient diarrhoea, dizziness, rash or muscular pains. As with other drugs the nurse will report any untoward symptoms.

De-Nol

This drug is taken orally, the dose being 5mls diluted in 15mls of water, to be taken four times daily as follows

Half an hour *before* the three main meals of the day.
One dose to be taken two hours *after* the last meal.
No liquids to be taken for at least half an hour *before* or half an hour *after* taking the drug.

The course of treatment lasts for 28 days and it is important that the drug is taken on an empty stomach. Milk should not be drunk during De-Nol treatment but the usual small amount taken in tea or coffee is allowed. Unlike other forms of therapy, antacids are *not* ordered as these may interfere with the action of the drug. Patients are strongly advised to take the medicine for the full course of treatment, even though relief from pain may have been achieved in a few days. De-Nol acts by coating the ulcer site and thus forming a protective layer against the action of gastric juices.

Presentation

De-Nol is presented in treatment packs which contain sufficient medicine for the four week course. The manufacturers also supply a leaflet giving the patient instructions.

Tagamet

Tablets   Syrup   Ampoules

200 mgms three times daily
400 mgms at night
The dose may be
increased

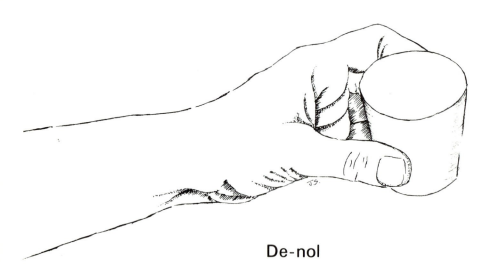

De-nol

5 mls in 15 mls of water
Half hour before three main daily meals
& two hours after last meal

Side effects

It may be noticed that the stools become discoloured or blackened during treatment.

Following a period under the above regimen, ulcers will heal but can recur. The patients are advised on discharge to eat small regular meals, avoid worry and stress and give up smoking. Surgery would be indicated if:

1　The ulcers fail to heal or recur very frequently.
2　The symptoms indicate to the possibility of pyloric stenosis.
3　Perforation has occurred.
4　Severe haematemesis.
5　There is a possibility of malignant change.

Haemorrhage, perforation and pyloric stenosis are complications of peptic ulceration.

Lack of pancreatic enzymes
Fibrocystic disease
Pancreatitis
Carcinoma

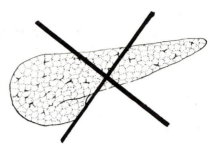

Lack of bile salts

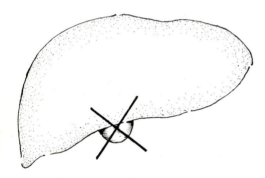

Biliary obstruction

Coeliac disease

Gluten induced
 enteropathy

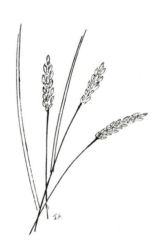

& Idiopathic steatorrhoea

4 Diseases of the intestine

Malabsorption

The main function of the intestine is to break down food substances into small molecules and so facilitate absorption into the
blood. The malabsorption syndromes are due to a failure of the
small intestine to absorb the essential nutrients, and can be
likened to a state of starvation whereby the body is deprived of
essential nutrients particularly proteins and vitamins. The result
is chronic diarrhoea and malnutrition.

Causes

Deficiency of pancreatic enzymes causes poor absorption of fat.
Fibrocystic disease of the pancreas, pancreatitis or carcinoma
may also cause such a deficiency. Lack of bile salts as a result of
biliary obstruction could also be a contributory factor. Perhaps
the condition known as coeliac disease would be more familiar
to nurses, a disease caused by the protein, gluten, found in wheat
and rye, which in susceptible individuals damages the mucosa of
the small intestine. Many authorities now call the condition
gluten induced enteropathy rather than coeliac disease.

The two conditions which will be discussed here are coeliac
disease, and its adult counterpart idiopathic steatorrhoea, and
they will be discussed jointly.

S/S
General Undeenourishment In the child, coeliac disease manifests itself in the first three
Stunting of growth years of life. It will be noticed that the child is irritable,
Abdominal dist. fractious and fails to thrive, with growth consequently being
Chronic diarrhoea retarded. Due to the lack of absorbed iron an iron deficiency
Rickety changes in anaemia develops. The stools are rather bulky, tend to float in
the bone water, and are rather offensive.

Idiopathic steatorrhoea in the adult presents itself in an
insidious fashion with the onset of loss of weight, general weakness and a noticeable looseness of the stools. The diarrhoea is
more or less persistent but the stools can return to near normal
for short periods of time. During the acute phase the stools are
bulky, pale, frothy and contain an excess of fat. Similar to
coeliac disease, anaemia is a feature due to the malabsorption of
both iron and folic acid. Deficiency of iron causing anaemia of
the hypochromic microcytic type, or lack of absorbed B_{12} and
folic acid causing anaemia of the hyperchromic macrocytic
variety. Deficiency of other food nutrients such as vitamin K can
result in haemorrhagic tendencies, or deficiency of potassium
causing confusion, weakness and apathy.

Diagnosis

Amongst the tests which may be employed in confirming the
diagnosis would be.

1 Fat absorption.

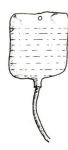

Correct electrolyte imbalance
and dehydration

Correct deficiency
of vitamins
& iron

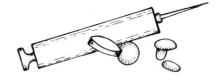

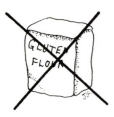

A low fat, high protein,
gluten free diet

Confirmed diagnosis is made by:—
a. Fat absorption test
b. Glucose tolerance test
c. Xylose tolerance test
d. Five day collection of
   stool specimens

4 Jejunal biopsy. [Crosby Capsule used to obtain specimen]

2 Glucose tolerance tests.

3 Xylose tolerance tests.

These tests enable the physician to distinguish between the steatorrhoea caused by malabsorption and the poor absorption of fat caused by disease of the pancreas.

Treatment of idiopathic steatorrhoea (Non Tropical Sprue)

associated with a Macrocytic type of anaemia.

Should there be evidence of dehydration with the possibility of electrolyte imbalance these will be corrected by intravenous infusion.

Deficiency of vitamins such as vitamin D, K or B are corrected accordingly, the anaemia being appropriately treated.

Specifically a gluten free diet is ordered, which initially may be easier to control when the patient is admitted. A diet low in fat and high in protein can also be ordered for certain patients.

The nursing care would include the collection of stool specimens over a period of five days and when diagnosis is confirmed ensuring strict adherence to the diet.

Regional ileitis or Crohn's disease will be discussed later, but other causes of malabsorption could include obstructive jaundice whereby in long standing cases the digestion of fats is impaired. Similarly lack of pancreatic enzymes in chronic pancreatitis will impair the digestion of both fat and protein resulting in steatorrhoea.

Tropical Sprue :— R₄ - Folic Acid.

Crohn's disease (regional ileitis)

This disease affecting mainly young people is one in which there are localised areas of chronic inflammation usually in the small intestine. The areas of small intestine involved undergo changes whereby the structure becomes thickened, oedematous and ulcerated, and thus become prone to secondary infection. The part of the intestine most commonly involved is the lower end of the ileum.

Clinical features

The patient usually complains of a colicky pain either in the region of the umbilicus, or perhaps centred in the right iliac fossa. The pain is often associated with a somewhat mild attack of diarrhoea.

Other features of the condition are:

Low grade pyrexia.

Loss of weight.

General weakness.

Moderate anaemia.

Raised ESR

The usual pattern is one of a gradual onset of the symptoms with long remissions, consequently the history will extend over a number of years. The condition is diagnosed by the physician palpating a tender mass in the right iliac fossa and by rectal

Regional ileitis

Colicky pain

Weight loss

Anaemia

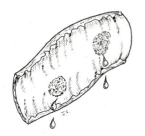

Anaemia

Diarrhoea

Low grade pyrexia

Raised E.S.R.

Treatment

Rest Physical & psychological

Diet Low residue, high protein
added vitamins

Drugs Steroids & to control
infections

Complications

Bowel stenosis

Fistulae

Perforation

Fistula in ano

Perianal abscess

examination. A barium meal will show the ulceration of the intestinal mucosa and possibly evidence of narrowing of sections of the gut.

Treatment

Initially the patient will be confined to bed, which in severe cases may be for a prolonged period, in order to ensure possibly both mental and physical rest. The patient must be given reassurance and kept free from worries or emotional problems.

The diet will be of low residue but of high protein content together with vitamin supplements because, as in other malabsorption states, these tend to be deficient.

Drugs used are the steroids and drugs such as pthalylsulphathiazole which may be of assistance in overcoming secondary infections present.

Complications of the disease include stenosis of the bowel, perforation and the formation of fistulae, perianal abscess or fistula in ano. Surgery may be required for some of the above particularly if obstruction or perforation occurs.

The nursing care will include all the routine duties plus the necessary observation of the patient for the onset of the more serious complications such as perforation or obstruction.

Ulcerative colitis

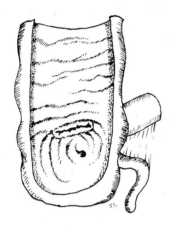

First affects
rectum &
extends to
ileo caecal
valve

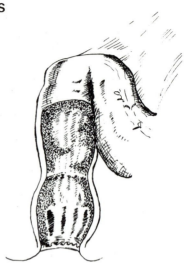

Signs & symptoms

Diarrhoea ⟶ Blood ⟶ Pus ⟶ Mucus

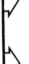 Pyrexia

 Anaemia

 Tachycardia

 Loss of weight

 Leucocytosis

5 Ulcerative colitis

The cause of this distressing, serious and chronic disease is unknown. Theories that it may be an auto-immune condition, or that the disease is due to psychological factors have been considered. It does appear that psychological influences are in some way contributory, inasmuch that psychological trauma such as the death of a loved one, or broken engagement can certainly cause a relapse in someone already suffering with the disease.

The disease first affects the rectum then spreads along the mucosa to involve the rest of the colon and may even involve the last part of the ileum. The mucous membrane becomes swollen, congested and bleeds rather easily, the colon eventually becoming ulcerated.

Clinical features

The disease usually starts in early adult life, the age bracket being between 20–40 years with little sex differentiation. The onset is usually insidious, the primary symptom being diarrhoea with blood and mucus in the stools. The attacks occur at intervals and during an acute phase there is an increase in the number and frequency of the stools. The patient will complain that prior to the passage of stools he feels a degree of pain and discomfort in the abdomen. A feature of this disease is that it can vary in severity ranging from a mild attack to a much more severe episode.

The patients will present with the following signs and symptoms:
Pyrexia, which will vary with the severity of the condition.
Anaemia, which can also be somewhat severe.
Tachycardia, either moderate or severe.
Loss of weight, sometimes proceeding to an emaciated condition.
The blood picture in addition to confirming the anaemia, will also show a degree of leucocytosis.

Nursing care

As there is no *specific treatment* the supportive measures which the nurse can offer will be beneficial to the patient and rewarding to the nurse.

Firstly she should ensure that the patient does have complete bed rest. The choice of bed should be one near the sluice in order that toilet demands can be speedily effected. A commode at the bedside will give the patient some degree of confidence when the need for a bedpan is urgent because frequent calls to stool are extremely distressing. The anal area will be very sore consequently care with anal toilet will do something for the patients comfort. He will also be distressed due to the offensive smell of the stool and a deodorant discreetly placed may help.

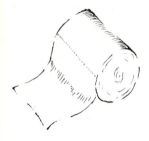

Frequent demand for bedpans.
Handwashing facilities
Soothing applications to
anal area

Poor appetite
Encourage intake of protein
& low residue foods

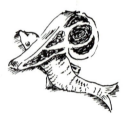

Iron for anaemia
Codeine phosphate & tincture of
opium.
Steroids.
Prednisolone retention enema.

Replacement of lost electrolytes
e.g.
Potassium
Sodium

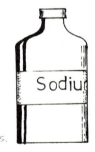

The sufferer can be very exhausted and weak, consequently gentle help in and out of bed will be required. As these patients are frequently fastidious people the nurse must be sure to *always* have a bowl of water nearby for hand washing after toilet, and to wash the patients hands if he appears too exhausted to do this for himself.

Consideration should also be given to any padding of bedpans when the patient is emaciated, likewise ensure that the bed is comfortable and well made. When the patient is confined to bed, the almost incessant demand for bedpans is wearing on the nurse but she must never indicate that the task is in any way irksome.

The pressure areas must be regularly attended to with particular care being taken when the patient is emaciated as the frequent passage of very loose stools makes the anal area very sore. Gentle washing with the application of a barrier cream may offer some comfort to the patient.

Diet
Many patients will not feel like eating, but with encouragement from the nurse a sufficiency of protein may be eaten. This is an important part of the diet because protein is lost in the stools and if not adequately replaced the patient will obviously have a protein deficiency. The diet given to the patient will be of low residue and may be presented in stages, commencing with a very light diet and progressing to one of a more substantial nature.

Medical treatment
It has been mentioned that there is no *specific* treatment for the disease but measures to raise the haemoglobin level will, when necessary, be undertaken. A blood transfusion may be given in severe cases together with iron, the drug being given parenterally if the oral route results in any further aggravation of the diarrhoea.

Drugs such as codeine phosphate or tincture of opium can also be ordered in an effort to control the diarrhoea.

Salazopyrin (Sulphasalazine) in doses of two grams daily may be ordered or the physician may request systemic steroid therapy. Prednisone or Prednisolone appear to be the drugs of choice. Retention enemata of Prednisolone hemisuccinate are sometimes ordered and can afford great relief to the patient.

The loss of potassium and sodium by the patient will be considered by the physician and be replaced in order to maintain the necessary levels in the blood. The patients electrolytes can be seriously upset.

Records
In addition to the routine TPR and blood pressure charts the nurse will be able to materially assist in the overall management of the patient if accurate records of the frequency of the diarrhoea are kept. This may enable the doctor to estimate losses of blood and fluid from the body.

Investigations

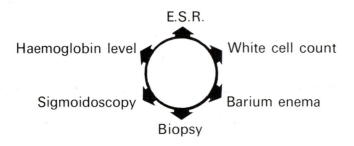

E.S.R.

Haemoglobin level · White cell count

Sigmoidoscopy · Barium enema

Biopsy

Complications

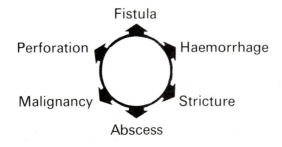

Fistula

Perforation · Haemorrhage

Malignancy · Stricture

Abscess

Surgical Treatment

Total colectomy

Formation of ileostomy

A very severe case of ulcerative colitis will tax both the skill of the medical practitioner as well as that of the nurses, the patient needing all the reassurance, support and encouragement that the ward team can give. The treatment given will often produce a remission but will not effect a cure.

Investigations
Blood tests for estimation of haemoglobin level and white cell count which will show both anaemia and leucocytosis.

ESR which will be raised.

Sigmoidoscopy, which may be omitted in the very ill patient.

Biopsy of the rectal mucosa.

Barium enema, this investigation too may be omitted in the severe case because it may cause perforation.

Complications
The condition can result in acute complications.
1 Perforation of the bowel leading to peritonitis.
2 Haemorrhage.
3 Recto-vesical fistula.
4 Malignant change.
5 Peri-anal abscess.
6 Stricture of the bowel.

Surgical treatment
Emergency surgery is indicated if certain complications arise e.g. perforation or stricture. In a proportion of cases, after due consideration, a total colectomy is performed in which case the terminal ileus is brought to the surface of the skin (Ileostomy). The intestinal contents are much more fluid and will present initial problems for all, but with the modern varieties of ileostomy appliances available many patients lead normal lives with a minimum of disability and are also able to take part in many physical activities.

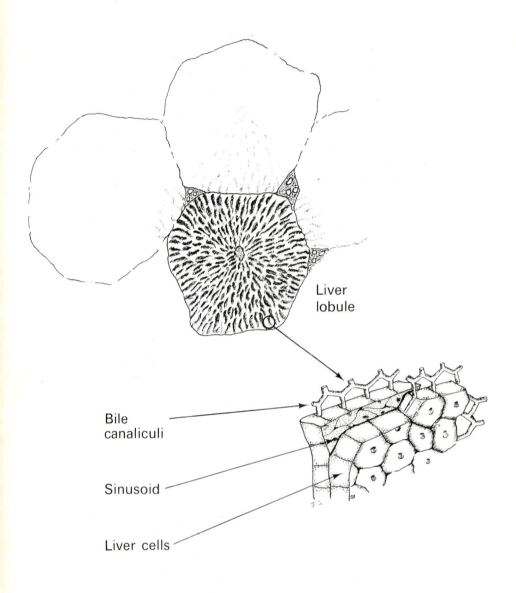

Liver
lobule

Bile
canaliculi

Sinusoid

Liver cells

Serum bilirubin — normal range
3·5 — 14 mmol/l per litre

6 Jaundice

Jaundice is the term given to the yellow discoloration of the skin and sclerae, and will be familiar to most nurses. It is very often the predominating sign in many diseases of the liver and biliary tract and is due to the increase in the serum bilirubin content of the blood above the normal range of 0.2–0.8mgms/mls (3.5–14.0 μ/mol per litre).

Jaundice as a clinical sign is usually apparent when the level of serum bilirubin is above 2 mgms% (35 μ/mol/litre) and the discoloration can be seen in the sclera, skin and mucous membrane. It may be of benefit, if before discussing causes of jaundice, a brief review of the liver and biliary tract is presented.

Bile is produced by the liver cells from the constituents of the blood. The cells of the lobules of the liver are arranged in rows – the liver cords radiating from a central vein. One side of the liver cord is exposed to the blood in the hepatic sinusoids, which is a mixture of both arterial blood from the hepatic artery, and blood from the portal vein. On the other side of the liver cord is a fine canal – the biliary canaliculus. The bile is formed by the cells from the constituents of the blood and discharged into the canaliculi which, eventually, by a series of ever increasing vessels drains into the hepatic ducts. The right and left hepatic duct unite to form the common hepatic duct and following storage in the gall bladder is discharged into the common bile duct and so into the duodenum at the ampulla of Vater.

Physiology of bile

After a life span of about 120 days the erythrocytes are broken down by elements of the reticulo endothelial system i.e. the spleen, Kupffer cells of the liver and also by the bone marrow.

The haemoglobin of the red blood cells is split into its iron component which is returned to the bone marrow for further use and into the iron free portion from which the pigment bilirubin is derived. On reaching the liver the bilirubin is changed from being insoluble to the soluble form which is present in the bile reaching the duodenum.

Bile, it will be recalled, is necessary for the breakdown and absorption of fats and also for the normal colour of faeces. It is the conversion of bilirubin into stercobilinogen in the intestines which is responsible for the normal colour of faeces. A certain amount of stercobilinogen is reabsorbed from the small intestine and returned to the liver via the portal vein, and discharged again as bile. The small amount under normal circumstances which escapes into the general circulation is excreted by the kidneys as urobilinogen.

Obstructive Jaundice

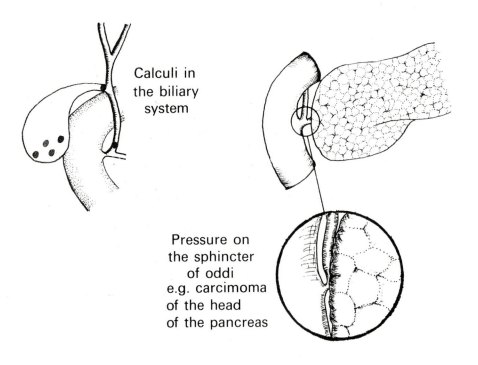

Calculi in
the biliary
system

Pressure on
the sphincter
of oddi
e.g. carcimoma
of the head
of the pancreas

Hepatic Jaundice

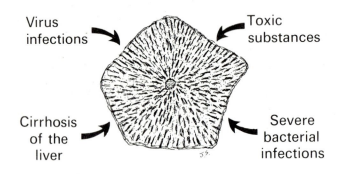

Virus
infections

Toxic
substances

Cirrhosis
of the
liver

Severe
bacterial
infections

Causes of jaundice

Jaundice can arise when too little bilirubin is removed from the blood in its passage through the liver which obviously raises the level of circulating bilirubin, or too much is liberated into the blood stream by an excessive breakdown of red blood corpuscles. The three main causes of jaundice are usually considered under the following headings.

1 Obstructive.
2 Hepatic.
3 Haemolytic.

Obstructive causes

Causes of obstructive jaundice are classed as being extra-hepatic when the obstruction occurs within the main bile ducts, or intra-hepatic where the lesion would be within the liver i.e. between the cells and the main bile ducts.

Conditions which come under the heading of extra-hepatic include gall stones within the common bile duct, carcinoma of the head of the pancreas or stricture of the bile duct.

Intra-hepatic causes include the jaundice caused by certain drugs and also as a result of diseases which damage the liver cells e.g. infective hepatitis. Many of the causes of obstructive jaundice are treated surgically by relieving the obstruction.

Whatever the cause of the obstruction, the jaundice is caused by the obstruction creating a back pressure which forces bile into the small lymphatic vessels surrounding the liver lobules and subsequently into the blood. The presence of the extra bilirubin thus raising the level of serum bilirubin above the threshold of 35 μ/mol/l resulting in the clinical features of jaundice.

Hepatic causes

In this type of jaundice the power of the liver cells to transfer bilirubin from the blood to the biliary canaliculi is reduced. The cells may be damaged by toxic substances or infective agents, the resulting degenerative processes permitting bilirubin which has entered the bile canaliculi to diffuse into the blood. Causes of jaundice under the above heading include:

1 Virus infections: infective hepatitis or serum hepatitis.
2 Toxic substances: drugs such as sulphonamides, PAS, Isoniazid and others. Poisons: carbon tetrachloride, chloroform and others.
3 Severe infections: septicaemia.
4 Cirrhosis of the liver.

Haemolytic causes

The increased rate of red blood corpuscle destruction will obviously result in increased bilirubin production. The normal healthy liver can adequately cope with a heavy load of extra bilirubin without jaundice being evident which is why in

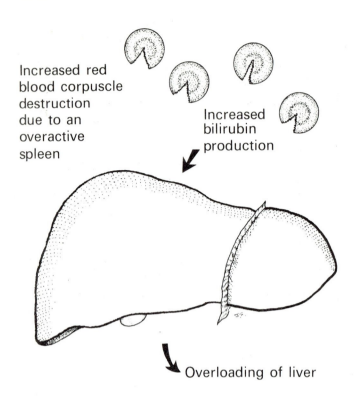

Increased red blood corpuscle destruction due to an overactive spleen

Increased bilirubin production

Overloading of liver

resulting in **Haemolytic Jaundice**

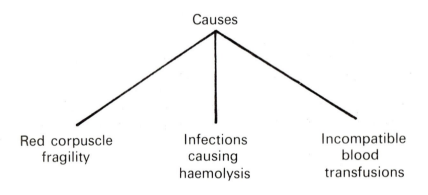

Causes

Red corpuscle fragility

Infections causing haemolysis

Incompatible blood transfusions

haemolytic jaundice, except in the newborn, the yellow discoloration is comparatively mild. Conditions which result in haemolytic jaundice include:

1 Fragility of red blood corpuscles due to congenital defects e.g. sickle cell anaemia.
2 Infections which cause excessive haemolysis.
3 Incompatible blood transfusions.

Clinical features

In discussing the clinical features, obstructive and hepatic jaundice will be considered separately because there are certain differences of significance in the haemolytic type. Viral causes will also be discussed under a separate heading.

Obstructive jaundice

1 Yellow discoloration of the sclera and skin, the discoloration often being first noticed in the sclerae.
2 The stools are pale due to the absence of stercobilinogen, bulky and foul smelling due to the presence of undigested fat.
3 The urine is dark due to the presence of bilirubin. The urine does NOT contain urobilinogen because none is absorbed from the small intestine.
4 Anorexia, nausea vomiting and an instinctive dislike of fatty foods.
5 Pruritis or skin irritation due to the presence of bile salts.
6 A slow pulse, again probably due to an excess of circulating bile salts.
7 A tendency to bleed due to the diminished absorption of vitamin K causing a fall in the prothrombin level of the blood.
8 A feeling of depression and irritability.

As indicated earlier certain forms of obstructive jaundice are amenable to surgery. The tendency to bleed can be reduced by giving vitamin K by injection and the skin irritation somewhat relieved by applying calamine lotion to the skin. Oral toilet will also assist in making the patient feel more comfortable. Glucose drinks are also of benefit.

Virus Hepatitis

Virus (probably in faeces)

Enters by oral route

Incubation 20–40 days

Symptoms

Headache	Anorexia	Jaundice	Malaise
Abdominal pain	Pyrexia	Pale stools	Dark urine
Nausea	Vomiting	Itchy skin	Depression

Treatment — none specific

Rest in bed until

Temperature subsides
Urine & stools return to
normal pattern
Appetite returns

Diet

High glucose content

Nursing care

Hygiene & handwashing

Convalescence is prolonged
Avoid alcohol

7 Viral hepatitis

Infective hepatitis

The cause of infective hepatitis is a virus probably spread by human faeces. The mode of entry is by oral means. The condition may arise as an epidemic in closed communities by direct personal contact, or perhaps spread by a healthy carrier.

The incubation period is about 20 to 40 days the patient presenting the symptoms of headache, malaise plus a degree of pyrexia. Other symptoms would be anorexia, nausea and vomiting. The abdominal pain experienced is non colicky in nature, the pain being the effect of the liver enlarging and so stretching the peritoneum. The patient will also exhibit the clinical features of jaundice such as pale stools, itchy skin, dark urine together with a degree of depression and irritability. Pulse is slow in relation to the degree of pyrexia present.

Treatment

There is NO specific treatment for infective hepatitis.

Generally the patient is kept in bed until the temperature subsides. The period of rest is continued until the appetite returns and the urine and stools return to a more normal pattern.

Initially the diet should have a high glucose content but the patient should be given whatever diet he fancies. Nurses and others who have to care for the patient should take great care in the disposal of excreta and pay particular attention to hand-washing after attending to any of the patients needs.

The convalescence is sometimes prolonged and all patients should be warned to avoid alcohol for three to four months following recovery. Most patients gradually recover over a period of three to six weeks.

Serum hepatitis

The main difference between infective hepatitis and serum hepatitis is in the mode of infection and the incubation period.

The virus is usually associated with the Australian antigen in the blood of certain individuals. It is transmitted by injections from inadequately sterilised needles, or from transfusions. It is because certain people have the virus in their blood that they are debarred from being blood donors. The incubation period is between 60 to 160 days.

Great care is taken in haemodialysis units in order to prevent any possibility of serum hepatitis occurring. This is an extremely serious condition requiring strict barrier nursing. The personnel in the unit being screened for Australian antigens.

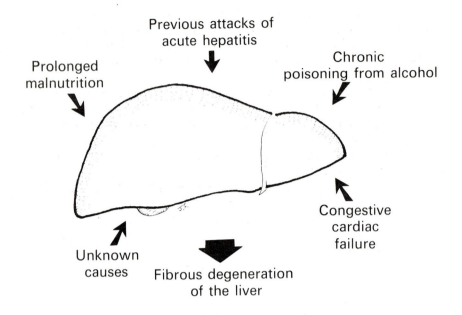

Previous attacks of
acute hepatitis

Prolonged
malnutrition

Chronic
poisoning from alcohol

Unknown
causes

Congestive
cardiac
failure

Fibrous degeneration
of the liver

Cirrhosis

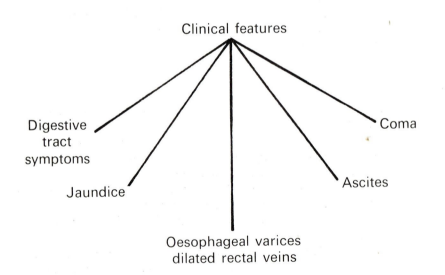

Clinical features

Digestive
tract
symptoms

Jaundice

Oesophageal varices
dilated rectal veins

Ascites

Coma

8 Haemolytic jaundice

Excessive destruction of red blood cells will manifest itself by causing both anaemia and jaundice although the jaundice may be comparatively mild. There are however certain differences between jaundice from obstructive causes and haemolytic causes.

1 The urine contains an excess of urobilin and will appear darker, particularly if left to stand.
2 The stools retain their normal colour or may even be a little darker.
3 The skin does not itch because there is no accumulation of bile salts in the blood.
4 As the liver can cope with an excess of bilirubin the jaundice may be slight or even absent in mild cases.
5 The conditions which produce haemolytic jaundice will obviously cause anaemia and are therefore discussed under haemolytic anaemias.

The treatment will be that of the cause.

Cirrhosis of the liver

In this chronic disease, fibrous degeneration of the liver occurs. It is a condition of multiple aetiology and can result from:

1 Previous attacks of acute hepatitis e.g. infective hepatitis or serum hepatitis.
2 Chronic poisoning from prolonged alcohol intoxication.
3 Malnutrition over a prolonged period.
4 Congestive cardiac failure.
5 Unknown.

Clinical features

1 The patient will complain of various symptoms associated with the digestive tract. Flatulence, nausea, anorexia and possible vomiting. He may also complain of pain in the right hypochondrium particularly following a meal.
2 Jaundice which may be variable in onset.
3 Oesophageal varices which can result in haematemesis, or also possible bleeding from dilated veins in the rectum.
4 Ascites which can arise as the cirrhotic condition of the liver progresses.
5 Coma due to the accumulation of certain nitrogenous compounds in the blood. The onset of coma may be preceded by severe mental changes which will result in an abnormal behaviour pattern in the patient.

Treatment

The diet will contain a high glucose content and be low in fat. Due to the possible accumulation of harmful nitrogenous com-

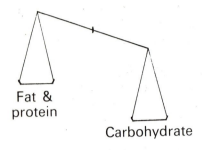

Fat & protein

Carbohydrate

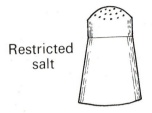

Restricted salt

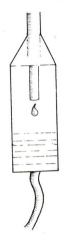

Intravenous infusion of dextrose / saline

Transfusion if bleeding occurs

Diuretics for ascites with potassium supplements

Treatment may include surgery: portacaval anastomosis

pounds, protein will be reduced to a minimum. Salt is restricted. Haematemesis can be of serious significance both from the loss of blood and because the digestion of the blood in the stomach will have the same result as giving the patient an increase in protein diet.

An intravenous infusion of dextrose/saline is often ordered but when bleeding from oesophageal varices or severe melaena occurs, then a blood transfusion is ordered. Persistent bleeding may need the introduction of a Sengstaken tube or even emergency surgery.

Ascites is usually controlled by very careful use of diuretics, hypokalaemia being prevented by the administration of potassium supplements.

After careful assessment certain patients are treated by surgery i.e. a porta-caval shunt whereby the portal vein is anastomosed to the inferior vena cava. This operation allows for the shunting of venous blood from the digestive system directly into the systemic circulation thus bypassing the liver.

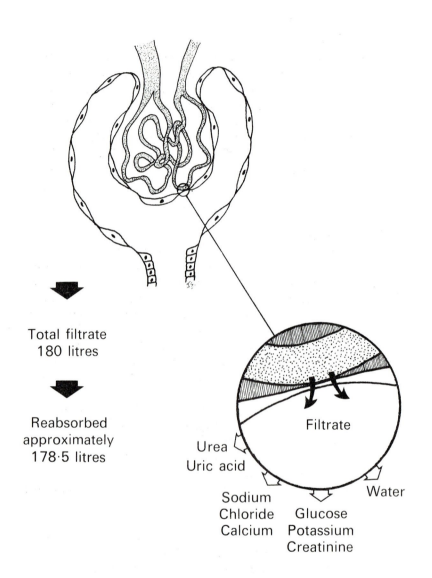

Total filtrate
180 litres

Reabsorbed
approximately
178·5 litres

Urea
Uric acid

Filtrate

Sodium
Chloride
Calcium

Glucose
Potassium
Creatinine

Water

9 The renal system

The functional unit of the kidney is the nephron and each kidney contains approximately one million. The nephron consists of:

1 The glomerulus.
2 The tubule.

The glomerulus or glomerular tuft is a mass of about fifty separate capillaries in a series of loops which fit into the upper expanded portion of the tubule i.e. Bowman's capsule.

The tubule follows a somewhat tortuous course and dips down into the medulla of the kidney finally emptying its contents into the collecting tubule. The walls of the Bowman's capsule are formed of a very thin membrane composed of a single layer of flat cells.

Tubular function

Each nephron is supplied with blood directly from the renal artery. The blood vessel leading into the capsule is the afferent arteriole which divides into a number of capillaries. The vessel leaving is the efferent arteriole which in turn forms a capillary network around the convoluted tubule eventually ending as a branch of the renal vein. Reference to the diagram will show that the blood is separated from the cavity of Bowman's capsule by the thin membrane of the capsule and the equally thin capillary walls. It is at this point that the first stage of urine formation takes place.

The pressure of blood forces water and dissolved substances in the plasma into Bowman's capsule but the cells and proteins are held back. As the operative force appears to be that of the blood pressure the need for a constant pressure to maintain glomerular filtration is obvious.

The glomerular filtrate consists of water and other substances such as:

Glucose	Sodium	Chloride	Urea
Potassium	Uric acid	Creatinine	Calcium

It has been estimated that about 180–200 litres of fluid are formed in 24 hours, or around 120 mls every minute. The amount of fluid passing through the glomerulus can be measured and is known as the Glomerular Filtration Rate (GFR). This test is an important indicator of kidney function.

The cells lining the tubules will selectively reabsorb various constituents required by the body, but allow to pass out any excess of electrolytes, waste products of metabolism, and water, thus maintaining the composition of body fluids at a constant level.

85% of water reabsorption
takes place in the proximal tubule

The antidiuretic hormone (A.D.H.)
exerts its action on the distal
tubule.

Reabsorption

Water: The amount of filtrate already mentioned, is about 180–200 litres a day but as urine passed is 1–2 litres daily then by far the greater percentage of water must be reabsorbed. About 85% of this water is reabsorbed by the proximal tubule but further absorption takes place in the distal tubule. It is at the distal tubules that the antidiuretic hormone from the posterior lobe of the pituitary gland exerts its action. When the plasma contains too much water less ADH is released, and therefore more water is allowed to pass out as urine. It will be recalled that certain diuretics (e.g. Frusamide) act at this point. Conversely when fluid is required to be retained by the body more ADH is released and less urine passed.

Sodium: The amount of sodium and chloride reabsorbed is carefully adjusted by the tubules in order that the total amount in the body remains constant. The proximal tubule is responsible for about 80% of the process. Hormonal control of sodium reabsorption comes from aldosterone secreted by the cortex of the adrenal gland. Aldosterone will increase tubular activity by raising the absorption of sodium and increasing the excretion of potasisum, being particularly active when the blood flow to the kidney falls.

Summary of the main functions of the kidney
1 To maintain the normal composition of plasma by excreting excess water and the waste products of metabolism e.g. urea, uric acid and creatinine.
2 To retain the essential constituents of the blood e.g. proteins, glucose and inorganic salts.
3 To regulate the acid base balance of the body by maintaining the tissue fluids at a constant composition thus assisting in the maintenance of the pH of tissue fluid.

Hormones produced by the kidney
It may be of interest to recall that the kidney also produces hormones. Angiotensin plays an important role in the control of blood pressure by its constricting effect on the arterioles.

Erythropoietin assists in the production of red blood cells.

Disease of the kidney consequently can affect both blood production and blood pressure.

A reduction, due to disease, of the amount of erythropoietin can result in a degree of anaemia, and an increase in the release of angiotensin cause an increase in blood pressure.

Urine

Specific gravity — 1,010 to 1,030   pH — 6·0

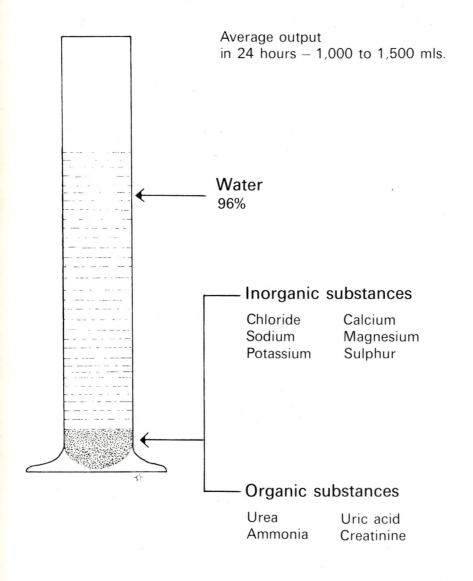

Average output
in 24 hours — 1,000 to 1,500 mls.

Water
96%

Inorganic substances

Chloride	Calcium
Sodium	Magnesium
Potassium	Sulphur

Organic substances

| Urea | Uric acid |
| Ammonia | Creatinine |

47

10 Urine

Normal constituents

As indicated previously, urine has a pH of about 6.0 but this will vary under dietary influences. Factors which will increase urinary acidity include a high protein diet, but so will starvation. Nurses may have noticed that diabetic patients often produce urine in which the acidity is raised. The specific gravity ranges between 1,010 to about 1,030 but in health will vary depending upon fluid intake. High fluid intake will obviously decrease the specific gravity just as a very low fluid intake will increase the specific gravity.

Volume

The output of urine is usually between 1,000–1,500 mls in 24 hours but again will depend upon fluid intake and also fluid loss via the skin, bowel and lungs. Excessive sweating from whatever cause will affect the output of urine secreted by the kidneys, just as patients with diarrhoea and vomiting will also have a reduced urinary output.

More urine is formed during the day than at night during sleep, excess urinary output during the night may be an early sign of chronic renal disease.

Composition of urine

Inorganic substances

Chloride	900 mgms per 100 mls 9 gms per litre.
Sodium	400 mgms per 100 mls 4 gms per litre.
Potassium	200 mgms per 100 mls 2 gms per litre.
Calcium	)
Magnesium	) in smaller amounts.
Sulphur	)

Organic or nitrogenous substances

Urea. The end product of protein metabolism.
Ammonia. Made in the kidney.
Uric acid.
Creatinine. Derived from the breakdown of body (endogenous) protein.

Urea, as indicated above is produced by the breakdown of the protein in the diet (exogenous protein), consequently it will vary with the amount of protein taken in the diet. The level of urea in the blood is 0.03 mgm% but in urine it is 2% approximately of the total solids. This means that the kidney tubules have had to concentrate the urea about 60 times. The power of the kidney to concentrate is of importance in renal disease and consequently the level of urea in the blood is of some significance. The normal range is 15–40 mgms%. Most nurses are aware that urine consists

Abnormal Constituents

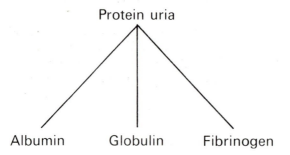

Protein uria

Albumin   Globulin   Fibrinogen

Causes of haematuria

Inflammation	Acute nephritis Pyelitis Cystitis Tuberculosis
Neoplasms	Hypernephroma Papilloma of the bladder
Embolism	Subacute bacterial endocarditis
Calculi	
Other causes	Trauma Prostatic conditions Overdose of anticoagulants

of water 96% salts 2% urea 2%, the above table simply breaks down the inorganic and organic substances in a little more detail.

It may be of interest to recall that in 24 hours 180 litres of water pass through the tubules of the kidney but as only 1.5 litres are passed out as urine the tubule must reabsorb 178.5 litres.

In health therefore the kidney must be able to selectively reabsorb essential substances and be able to maintain the acid base balance of the body. Any condition or disease which interferes with filtration in the glomerulus and with tubular function will result in possible widespread effects in the body and could result in abnormal urinary constituents.

Abnormal urinary constituents

Proteinuria: The discovery of protein in the urine indicates that albumin (the smallest protein molecule) and perhaps those of globulin and fibrinogen have leaked across the glomerular membrane. Nurses often speak of albumin in the urine but it is worthwhile remembering that other plasma proteins come under the title of proteinuria.

Proteinuria is usually, but not always, indicative of renal disease. Despite the simplicity of modern methods of urine testing it should still be undertaken with care because sometimes even a small but detectable amount may well be the first indication of a severe renal condition.

Haematuria: Blood in the urine can arise from (i) kidney, (ii) ureters, (iii) bladder. Blood from the kidney itself will be intimately mixed with urine and may be obvious or give the urine its 'smoky' appearance and will be positively identified on testing. There are many causes of haematuria, amongst which are:

1 Acute nephritis.
2 Hypernephroma.
3 Papilloma of the bladder.
4 Trauma.
5 Subacute bacterial endocarditis.
6 Pyelitis.
7 Cystitis.
8 Prostatic conditions.
9 Renal calculi.
10 Overdose of anticoagulants.
11 Tuberculosis of the renal tract.

As indicated blood in the urine can arise from a number of causes and usually indicates a possibly serious disease of the urinary tract. The examining physician or surgeon will always fully investigate the patient in order to discover the cause.

Pus cells: Inflammation of any part of the urinary tract may result in pus cells being present. When a specimen is sent for

Laboratory specimens of urine should be fresh. Specimens for culture are collected using aseptic techniques to avoid contamination.

Carry out ward urine testing on fresh specimens.

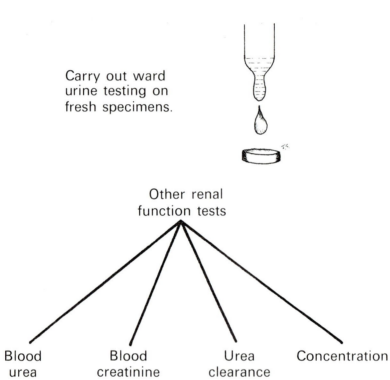

Other renal
function tests

| Blood urea | Blood creatinine | Urea clearance | Concentration |

culture the nurse must ensure that the specimen is fresh and sent to the laboratory immediately. In acute renal infections the urine will be cloudy and have the typical 'fishy' odour.

Bile and urobilinogen have been discussed on pages 32 and 34.

The testing of urine in the ward is an important nursing duty and one which should always be performed with care on freshly passed urine.

Other tests of renal function include:

1 Blood urea.
2 Blood creatinine.
3 Urea clearance test.
4 Concentration test.

An accurately maintained fluid chart will indicate oliguria, polyuria and anuria. Correct records of the amount of urine passed will indicate, inter alia, the concentration and excretory powers of the kidneys.

Acute nephritis

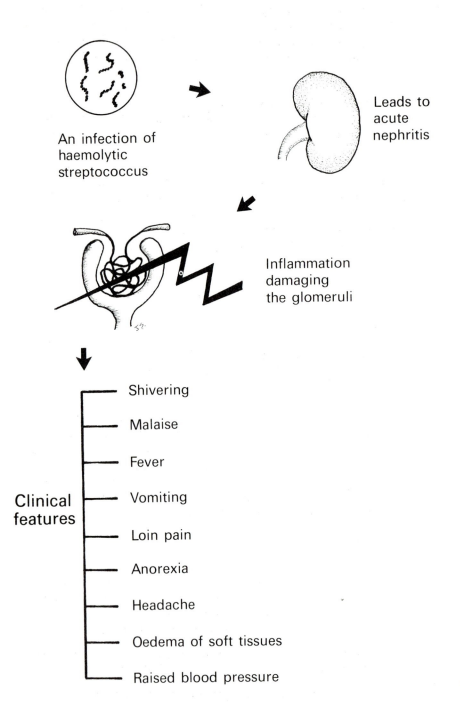

An infection of
haemolytic
streptococcus

Leads to
acute
nephritis

Inflammation
damaging
the glomeruli

Clinical
features

- Shivering
- Malaise
- Fever
- Vomiting
- Loin pain
- Anorexia
- Headache
- Oedema of soft tissues
- Raised blood pressure

11 Nephritis

There are many conditions affecting the kidneys which come under the heading of nephritis, and an exact classification presents difficulties. The disease may be defined as a bilateral, non-suppurative, diffuse disease of the kidneys, and only the more common conditions which may be encountered by the nurse will be discussed.

Acute nephritis (acute glomerulonephritis)

This condition occurs mostly in childhood or adolescence, can arise at any age, but now appears to be much less common than hitherto.

The usual pattern is that the onset of the disease follows a recent infection caused by the haemolytic streptococcus. The condition may consequently follow such infections as tonsillitis or scarlet fever which had been present two to three weeks previously. Present day thinking appears to support the theory that the disease is of immunological origin, that is, it is probably an allergic reaction to the previous haemolytic streptococcal infection and is due to antigen-antibody reaction resulting in damage to the glomerular membrane.

Pathology

The glomeruli of the kidney show certain inflammatory changes, the resultant damage to the glomeruli being responsible for such abnormalities as haematuria and proteinuria.

Clinical features

The onset is fairly sudden following the history indicated above, patients presenting with shivering, malaise, fever and vomiting. They may also complain of pain in the loins, anorexia and headache, other features of the disease are oedema of soft tissues particularly around the eyes giving the individuals face a rather puffy appearance and if the patient has been ambulant there could also be some oedema of the ankles. The blood pressure could show a moderate rise.

Urinary changes

Oliguria: There is an obvious reduction in urinary output and in severe cases the patient may be anuric. The reduced output is due to a reduction of glomerular filtration, because of the disease and also to an increase in tubular reabsorption.

Haematuria: The urine will be either smoky or may even be red due to the presence of varying amounts of blood.

Proteinuria: Protein is usually present but is not normally very high.

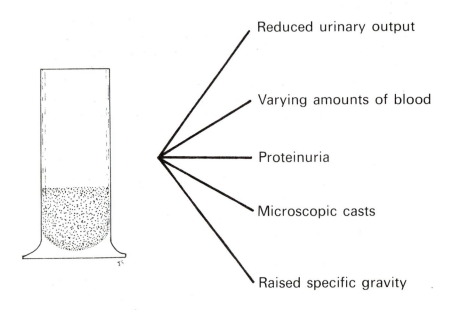

Reduced urinary output

Varying amounts of blood

Proteinuria

Microscopic casts

Raised specific gravity

Treatment

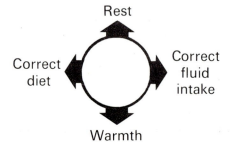

Rest

Correct diet

Correct fluid intake

Warmth

Casts: These are detected by microscopic examination.

Specific gravity: Raised.

Course and prognosis
About 90–95% of children make a complete recovery from this disease but the prognosis is not quite so favourable with adults over middle age. In patients who do not make a complete recovery the signs and symptoms persist with increasing evidence of renal failure, and death can result within one year. Other patients may apparently recover but continue to pass albumin in the urine and eventually develop nephrotic syndrome or chronic renal failure.

Treatment and nursing care
The aim of the treatment will be to maintain the patient until a spontaneous recovery of renal function occurs, which as indicated previously will happen with 90–95% of patients.

The nurses particular role will be to make sure the patient has adequate rest and warmth, the correct diet and correct fluid intake as instructed by the physician.

The patient will be nursed in a warm, draught free room, every effort being made to see that the patient does not suffer any chilling of the skin. Patients who completely recover are normally allowed up in 2–4 weeks when the haematuria, proteinuria and oedema have disappeared and the blood pressure is normal.

Dietary regulation
Many physicians consider a reduction of protein intake to be of value and will order a diet containing 20–40 gms of protein daily, but sufficient calories will be given in the form of carbohydrates and fats, obviously both salt and fluid will be restricted. Fluids may be restricted to 500–750 mls per day *plus* the previous days urinary output. The importance of an *accurately* kept fluid chart is obvious.

Diuresis usually occurs within a few days and when this happens the diet will be stepped up to include more protein. After a while the food intake is gradually increased to that of a normal diet.

The specific nursing observations will be:
1 Daily urine testing for protein and blood.
2 Daily urine volume.
3 Daily blood pressure.
4 Observation of temperature, pulse and respiration.

The nurse will be particularly observant for any severe headache, alteration of pulse rate and for the onset of diuresis.

During the early acute stage oral toilet, pressure area and skin care will assist in making the patient more comfortable.

Specific nursing duties in acute nephritis.

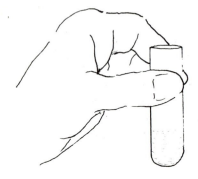

Urine testing daily
for
proteins
&
blood

Measurement &
recording of
daily urine
volume

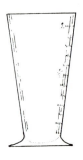

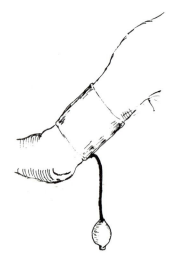

Measurement &
recording of
daily blood
pressure

Observation
of
temperature
pulse
respiration

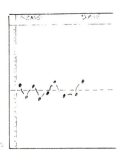

In the small percentage of cases which do not recover completely, albumin is always present in the urine and the blood pressure remains moderately raised. These patients will be diagnosed as subacute nephritis and will eventually be treated for chronic nephritis.

Elimination of infection
In order to eliminate foci of infection the patient will probably be ordered some form of penicillin for five days. Many physicians consider that children should be given an oral preparation of penicillin for a few years as a prophylactic measure. Infected tonsils or teeth which could have been the focus of infection will be removed following a suitable convalescent period.

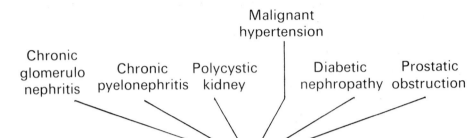

Malignant
hypertension

Chronic
glomerulo
nephritis

Chronic
pyelonephritis

Polycystic
kidney

Diabetic
nephropathy

Prostatic
obstruction

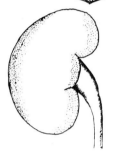

Chronic renal failure

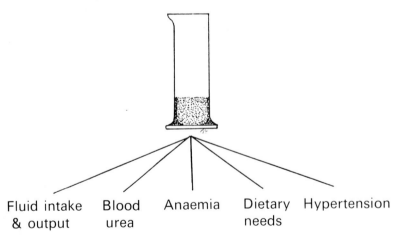

Fluid intake
& output

Blood
urea

Anaemia

Dietary
needs

Hypertension

12 Chronic renal failure

Chronic renal failure can be the end result of a large number of different diseases of the kidneys. Amongst such progressive and usually long standing diseases are:

1 Chronic glomerulo-nephritis.
2 Chronic pyelonephritis.
3 Polycystic kidney.
4 Malignant hypertension.
5 Diabetic nephropathy.
6 Prostatic obstruction.

It sometimes happens that the patient, in the early stages, is unaware that he has a disease of the kidneys; the condition being gradual in onset and perhaps only being discovered at some investigation. However, as the condition is progressive then symptoms of kidney failure such as polyuria, nocturia, raised blood pressure and proteinuria will appear. At this stage the blood urea may only be slightly raised the patient possibly complaining of lack of energy which will be due to a degree of anaemia.

Many patients with chronic renal failure can live for years by good management of diet, protein intake and fluid balance, but eventually the disease progresses to the advanced degree and is called uraemia. As there is no cure the treatment will be directed to making the patients life more tolerable by as far as possible relieving him of any discomfort.

The physician will be, inter alia, particularly interested in:

1 Fluid intake and output.
2 The level of blood urea.
3 Degree of anaemia.
4 Degree of hypertension.
5 Any dietary restrictions necessary.

The urine will be of a fixed specific gravity with the output usually increased, one nursing duty being to ensure that the fluid intake is relatively high (approximately 3 litres daily). The level of the blood urea will determine the amount of protein allowed. Blood urea of 16 mmols/l% and above will require a protein intake of 20–40 gms. Unless relieved by such measures as peritoneal or haemodialysis the condition will eventually lead to the toxic, fatal condition – uraemia.

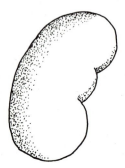

Chronic renal failure
results in:

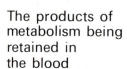

The products of
metabolism being
retained in
the blood

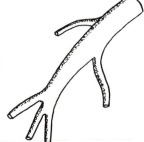

A reduced urinary output
of toxic substances

Uraemia

13 Uraemia

The causes and certain features of chronic renal failure have been mentioned on page 60 but eventually as kidney function progressively worsens, other symptoms become evident. One of the major effects will be hypertension which will in turn lead to still further renal damage.

Severe chronic renal failure is a condition whereby the patient is poisoning himself with the retained products of his own metabolism and may be classed as uraemic, the term uraemia literally meaning 'urine in the blood' and therefore implies that toxic substances are being retained e.g. urea.

Reference to the structure and function of the nephron will show that the amount of filtrate through the glomerulus is about 120 mls per minute which equals approximately 200 litres in 24 hours. Of this enormous amount of fluid passing through the tubules, only about $1\frac{1}{2}$ –2 litres are passed as urine. The amount of filtrate can be measured in a test known as the Glomerular Filtration Rate (GFR) and briefly the significance of this test is that it indicates the clearance of certain substances out of the blood. Obviously if the GFR becomes progressively lower then toxic substances are not cleared from the plasma and so stay in the blood.

When the kidneys progressively fail the effect on the individual will be widespread, and affect many systems of the body.

1 The pallor and anaemia of the patient is always a noticeable feature due possibly to a deficient production of erythropoietin. Additionally there appears to be an increase in the breakdown of red blood corpuscles as well as a deficiency of production. The degree of anaemia present is often compatible with the severity of the renal failure.

2 Anorexia and vomiting are common symptoms and the nurse will notice that the breath has an unpleasant odour. The foul state of the mouth will be an obvious indication for frequent oral toilet.

3 Dyspnoea and cyanosis can be troublesome for the patient and when combined with hiccoughs, which are often present, results in a very distressing feature of the disease.

4 Convulsions which can occur are due to the degree of hypertension present.

5 Heart failure due to hypertension and overloading of the circulation with an increased volume of water and salt.

Urinary output

The urinary output is large and of fixed specific gravity due to the lack of concentrating power of the kidney. Patients will also be noticed to pass more urine at night.

BLOOD PRESSURE.
TEMPERATURE
PULSE &
RESPIRATIONS.

ACCURATE
FLUID BALANCE
CHARTS.

RECORD
PATIENTS
WEIGHT.

24 HOUR
URINE
SPECIMEN

ORAL
TOILET

CARE WITH
ORDERED
DIETARY
INTAKE.

Other systems affected include the endocrine, skeletal and neuromuscular. Vision may be impaired the physician noting any papilloedema present. As with all conditions of severe acidosis the respirations will be slow and deep.

Nursing care

Routinely the temperature, pulse, respiration and blood pressure will be recorded but the frequency of such recordings will depend on whether or not the patient is in heart failure or severely hypertensive. An accurate fluid balance chart must be kept together with a record of the patients weight. Other nursing duties will include keeping a 24 hour specimen of urine. The diet will be especially ordered and the nurse will ensure that it is adhered to.

The nurse will note whether the patient is constipated, which can arise due to the large volume of fluid lost via the urine; there may be a tendency to dehydration.

The importance of oral toilet has been mentioned, and when regularly performed may make the severely ill patient feel a little more comfortable.

Medical treatment

The physician will inter alia consider the form of treatment most suitable for the particular patient taking also into account the cause of the renal failure. Urinary infections and hypertension will be treated with the appropriate drugs but drugs will be chosen with care as some patients will not be able to *effectively excrete* the drug.

Diet and fluid intake

Protein foods will be carefully selected in both type and amount in order to prevent any rise in the blood urea level. In severe chronic renal failure there is both a loss of water and salt and so the correct balance between intake and output will be maintained.

Any infection will be treated with antibiotics but as with other drugs they are chosen with care in view of the patients poor renal function.

Eventually the stage may be reached when the decision for dialysis will have to be made, a decision which is never an easy one for the medical officers concerned.

The nephrotic syndrome

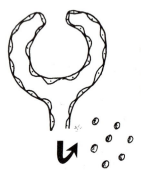

The damaged glomerulus
allows protein molecules
to pass

Albumin
&
globulin

Resulting in

Oedema

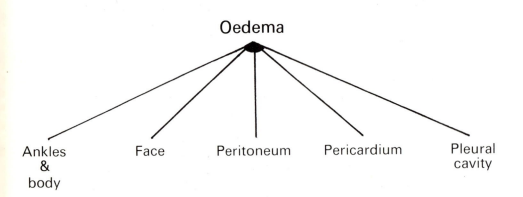

Ankles   Face   Peritoneum   Pericardium   Pleural
&   cavity
body

14 The nephrotic syndrome

There are many causes of the above condition amongst which would be:
1 Subacute glomerulonephritis.
2 Diabetic nephropathy.
3 Systemic lupus erythmatosus.

Pathology

The disease is characterised by an excessive loss of plasma proteins in the urine. The damaged glomerulus allows the molecules of albumin to pass through fairly easily but as the disease progresses there is also a loss of globulin which has a larger molecular structure.

The reduction in the plasma proteins in the blood due to this loss results in a lowered plasma osmotic pressure causing a diffusion of fluid into the tissue spaces and so resulting in oedema. The loss of fluid from the plasma to the tissues will obviously cause a fall in circulatory blood volume.

Clinical features

The onset of the nephrotic syndrome is insidious with the oedema being noticeable firstly in the ankles but gradually the oedema extends to the whole body. Fluid will collect in the peritoneum, pericardium and pleural cavities with the face presenting the typical pale and puffy appearance. The urine will contain large amounts of protein but at this stage the blood urea is normal. The cause of the disease depends upon the underlying cause and is somewhat variable. In the majority of cases renal failure develops and death occurs.

Treatment

The aim of the treatment is directed at the relief of the oedema and the reduction of the proteinuria.

Relief of oedema: As the patient is losing large quantities of protein in the urine and the blood urea is within normal limits a high protein diet is given. The patient should receive about 100 gms of protein daily, the normal diet being supplemented with protein drinks such as Complan. Salt will obviously be restricted. Diuretics such as Frusemide or Spironolactone are ordered, sometimes together, particularly when there has been a marked loss of potassium. On occasions mechanical drainage of the chest and abdomen are required.

Steroids such as Prednisolone are administered and most patients are given this form of treatment. When effective there is a marked improvement with a progressive decrease in the proteinuria and oedema. Steroid treatment is more effective with children than with adults.

Treatment of nephrotic syndrome

High protein diet
Restricted salt
Diuretics
Paracentesis abdominus
Steroids
Immuno-suppressive drugs

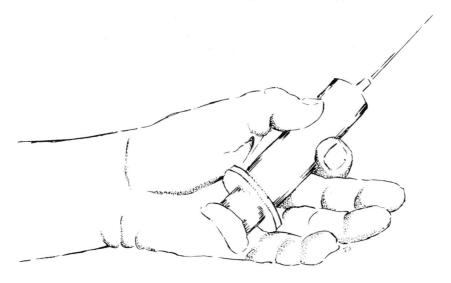

Care of pressure areas
Fluid balance chart
24 hour urine specimens
Encourage patient to take diet

With certain forms of nephrotic syndrome immuno-suppressive drugs such as Cyclophosphamide and Azothioprine are used.

Nursing care

Most patients are nursed at bed rest particularly when there is gross oedema but as the oedema responds to treatment they are allowed up.

As with all other conditions of oedema the pressure areas require constant attention in order to prevent any breakdown of the skin. In addition to the routine fluid chart, a 24 hour specimen of urine will be required in order to accurately assess the amount of protein lost daily. Nurse will try and encourage the patient to persist with the high protein and low salt diet which may not be very appetising.

Cystitis

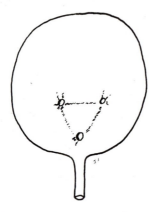

Causative organisms

| Escherichia coli | Proteus vulgaris | Streptococcus faecalis | Pseudomonas pyocyanous | Staphylococcus aureus |

Treatment

Sulphonamides
or
antibiotics

Frequent attacks require
urological investigation

15 Urinary tract infections

Cystitis
Cystitis is predominantly a disease of women, the short female urethra allowing bacteria from the perineum and related areas to spread to the bladder. The most common infecting organism is *Escherichia coli* but Proteus vulgaris, Streptococcus faecalis, Staphylococcus aureus and Pseudomonas pyocyaneous are also causative agents. It will also be recalled that unsterile catheterisation techniques can also be a contributory factor.

Clinical features
Frequency and pain on micturition are the main features of the condition which may be associated with uterine prolapse, or be precipitated by sexual intercourse (honeymoon cystitis).

If the sufferer is in hospital the nurse will be asked to obtain a midstream specimen of urine. Normal urine can contain up to 10,000 bacteria per millilitre but in urinary tract infections the figure will be appreciably increased i.e.± 100,000 per millilitre.

Treatment
The attack usually responds to a short course of sulphonamides or antibiotics but in repeated attacks the physician will consider a full urological investigation because the disease can give rise to pyelonephritis.

Pyelonephritis. Acute
The term pyelonephritis indicates that there is inflammation of mainly the ureters and pelvis of the kidney, but the infective process can also affect structures in the kidney.

Causes
  1 May follow an attack of cystitis.
  2 Urinary stasis:
     a bladder neck obstruction in males.
     b pregnancy.
     c blood borne infections.
     d congenital defects in children.
     e calculi.
  3 Neurological disorders i.e. those which interfere with complete emptying of the bladder.

Clinical features
  1 The onset is sudden with a marked pyrexia.
  2 Rigors may be present.
  3 General feeling of malaise.
  4 Frequency of micturition.
  5 Dysuria.

Acute pyelonephritis

Inflammation of the
kidney pelvis & ureter

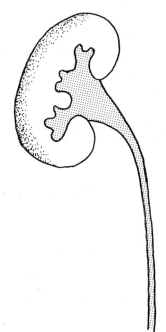

Causes

Cystitis
Urinary stasis
Neurological disorders

Clinical features

1. Pyrexia   2. Rigors   3. Malaise

4. Frequency   5. Dysuria   6. Loin pain

7. Pus cells in
the urine

6 There may be an aching pain in both loins.

7 The urine contains many pus cells.

Treatment and nursing care

The patient is put to bed in the position which he finds most comfortable. A urine specimen is obtained and sent for culture and sensitivity tests. Fluids are encouraged and if possible the patient will drink about three litres a day.

E. coli infections flourish in acid urine consequently treatment will be ordered to make the urine alkaline by giving the patient sodium citrate and sodium bicarbonate. The nurse will see that the patient takes the mixture as ordered and also test the urine frequently in order to determine when the urine becomes alkaline.

The sensitivity test will indicate the chemotherapeutic or antibiotic treatment which will of course be specific to the causative organism.

It is important that the infection is eradicated because persistent and recurrent attacks result in the chronic form of the disease.

Pyelonephritis. Chronic

Many patients will have a history of prolonged kidney infections but other cases do not present any relevant history.

The clinical features will be similar to those of the acute form but on occasions may also be the initial clinical features of renal failure, however when the diagnosis of chronic pyelone-phritis is confirmed then the aim of the treatment will be to eradicate the infection, which may take some time.

The investigation of the patient will include such investigations as intravenous pyelogram, cystoscopy, micturating cystogram and renal biopsy.

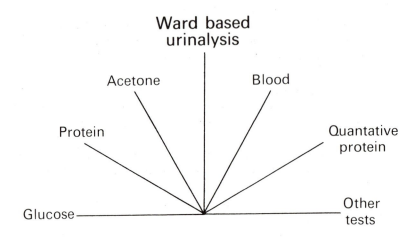

Ward based urinalysis

- Acetone
- Blood
- Protein
- Quantative protein
- Glucose
- Other tests

24 hour specimens laboratory tests

Concentration
1. Specific gravity
2. Concentration tests
3. Dilution tests

Bacteriological
1. M.S.U.

Blood
1. Electrolytes

Renal function
1. Glomerular filtration rate
2. Creatinine
3. Urea clearance

16 Renal investigations

There are many renal investigations which can be ordered, some of which will directly concern the nurse, but as with investigations for other diseases, a modicum of understanding will be of benefit in appreciating the treatment ordered.

1 Ward based urine tests
All nurses should be familiar with the tests for glucose, protein, acetone, blood etc., and also for the routine required for 24 hour specimens, and when ordered, the quantitative test for protein (Esbachs). Care and accuracy are required for all tests but the co-operation of the patient is required for some e.g. 24 hour specimens.

The simplicity of modern ward based tests for urinary abnormalities should not allow the nurse to forget that much can be learned from critical observation of the urine for colour, smell, turbidity and deposits. It may be of benefit if the senior nurse sometimes checks her junior colleagues in the routine testing of urine.

2 Tests for concentration
1. Specific gravity.
   normally 1,002–1,030.
2. Concentration tests.
   The particular nursing duty will be to see that the patient does not drink for about twelve hours. She may be asked to weigh the patient.
3. Dilution tests.
   Nursing duties are to give the required amount of water (1.5 litres) at the specific times and to see that the bladder is emptied at hourly intervals for four hours. Each hour the specific gravity and volume are recorded.

3 Bacteriological examination
1. MSU.

4 Tests on blood
1. Electrolytes.

5 Renal function
1. Glomerular filtration rate.
2. Creatinine.
3. Urea clearance.

6 X ray
1. Straight X ray of abdomen.
2. Intravenous pyelogram (IVP) or perhaps called the intravenous urogram (IVU).

Xray examinations
of the renal tract

Xray of abdomen

Intravenous pyelogram

Nursing duties

1. Give the prescribed aperient
2. Give low residue diet
3. Restrict fluids
4. Avoid enemata

Micturating cystogram
Nursing duties

1. Reassure & explain
2. Catheterise the patient
3. Send fresh specimen
   to laboratory

Nursing duties

a By giving the ordered aperient e.g. Senakot or Dulcolax the intestines are cleared of faeces or gas.

b Ensure that the low residue diet is free from vegetables, cereals or wholemeal bread.

c Restrict fluid as ordered.

d It is better to avoid enemata.

7 Micturating cystogram

The nurse can be of some assistance in this somewhat embarrassing test by giving the necessary explanation and reassurance. The specific nursing duty will be to catheterise the patient on the ward and send the specimen immediately to the pathological laboratory.

Other tests and investigations include renal biopsy and renal arteriograms.

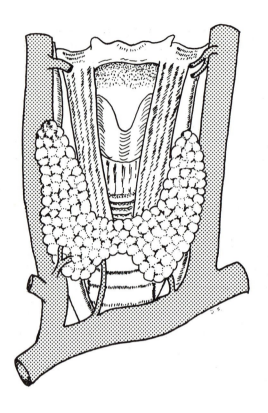

The thyroid gland

Consists of vesicles
lined with cuboid
epithelium containing
the thyroid hormones
which are released
into surrounding
blood vessels

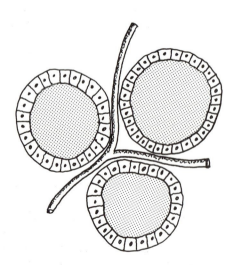

17 Thyrotoxicosis

Before proceeding with diseases of the thyroid gland, it may be of advantage to review briefly the anatomy and physiology of the gland itself. The gland consists of two lateral lobes, joined to each other by the isthmus. The blood supply is a rich one via both the superior and inferior thyroid arteries. The structure consists of vesicles which resemble closed spherical sacs, the sacs being lined with a single layer of cuboid epithelium. Each vesicle contains within it the colloid material in which can be found the active principles of the thyroid hormones. These iodine containing hormones are thyroxine and tri-iodothyronine, some of which is stored in the colloid which in turn releases a certain amount into the surrounding blood vessels and so into the circulation.

The control of thyroid activity is largely dependent upon hormones released by the anterior lobe of the pituitary gland namely the thyrotrophic hormone or thyroid stimulating hormone (TSH). The function of TSH is concerned with cellular metabolism, regulating the metabolic activities of tissues according to their varying needs. Excessive secretion of the thyroid hormone results in hyperthyroidism (thyrotoxicosis). An important nerve, the recurrent laryngeal nerve, is in close relationship to the thyroid gland and lies in the space between the trachea and the oesophagus.

Thyrotoxicosis
The condition is also known by other titles e.g. Graves's disease, toxic goitre and exophthalmic goitre. The condition appears to occur more frequently in women, the onset usually presenting in early adult life.

Aetiology
It has already been mentioned that over production of thyroxine can result in thyrotoxicosis but another substance called long acting thyroid stimulator (LATS) which is found in the plasma of thyrotoxic patients is also a contributory factor.

Clinical features
The patient often presents as a restless, nervous individual, with undue sweating. She also complains of tiredness and breathlessness on exertion together with palpitations and tachycardia. Patients often state that the temperature of a room that most people find satisfactory, is much too hot for them, and conversely that temperatures which the patient can tolerate are too cold for others.

On examination the doctor finds that the outstretched hands will show a fine tremor, other signs include:

Thyrotoxicosis
Clinical features

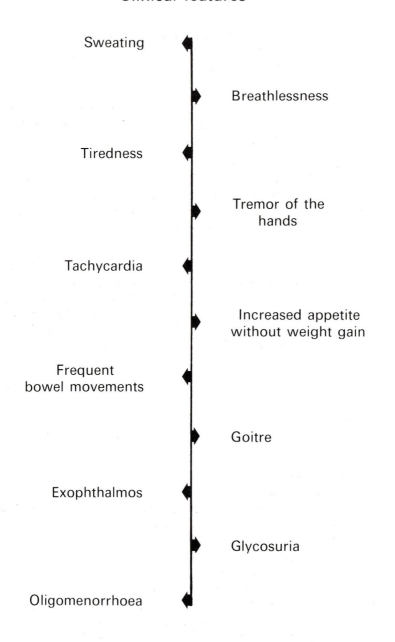

Sweating

Breathlessness

Tiredness

Tremor of the hands

Tachycardia

Increased appetite without weight gain

Frequent bowel movements

Goitre

Exophthalmos

Glycosuria

Oligomenorrhoea

1 Sinus tachycardia

A feature of the fast pulse rate is that it persists during sleep and one of the nursing duties therefore is on occasions to take the 'sleeping pulse'. The nurse may also find atrial fibrillation to be present.

2 Appetite

This is increased but if the increased metabolism is excessive then weight loss will occur. Nurses may be requested to keep a record of any weight loss or gain.

3 Bowels

Patients may also complain that there has been some change in their bowel habits i.e. they now pass loose stools or that they have to empty the bowel more frequently than previously.

4 Enlarged thyroid gland

This can be obvious but the physician may detect that the swelling is greater on one side than the other. It also happens that there is no detectable swelling due to the thyroid increasing in size retrosternally, and consequently is not so obvious.

5 Exophthalmos

The prominence of both eyes can be a striking feature of the condition and is due to the eyes being pushed forward. It is considered to be due to oedema behind the eyeball. It may also be observed that the patients upper eyelid cannot follow the movement of the eyeball when the patient looks down. This feature is termed 'lid lag'.

6 Glycosuria

On testing the urine a slight degree of glycosuria may be detected and should be reported.

7 Oligomenorrhoea

Oligomenorrhoea can occur in a reasonably large number of female patients.

Investigations

The disease can be confirmed by:

1 Radioactive isotopes 131 I which indicates that there is an increase in the uptake of iodine.
2 Serum protein bound iodine.
3 Tri-iodothyronine resin bound uptake, T3.
4 Thyroxine assay, T4.

The tests will measure the amount of organic iodine circulating in the blood in the form of thyroxine. When these tests are being performed the nurse can be of some assistance if she realises that the tests may be invalidated if any preparation containing iodine has been taken by the patient, perhaps in some diagnostic procedures. Other drugs particularly hormone preparations e.g. the contraceptive pill can influence the result by interfering with the test.

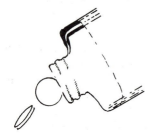

Treatment is
carbimazole tablets

or

Iodine   (I^{131})

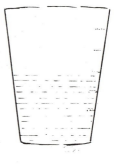

If carbimazole is
not tolerated **stop**
and give methyl thiouracil
and digoxin if atrial fibrillation
occurs

Nursing care includes
1. A quiet bed in the ward
2. T.P.R., apex beat & sleeping pulse
3. Daily bathing
4. Adequate diet & ample fluids
5. Watch for side effects of drugs

Treatment

The medical treatment of this condition is usually by the administration of antithyroid drugs such as Carbimazole or by using radioactive iodine 131 I. The physician will carefully consider many details before deciding upon the form of treatment suitable for the patient.

When Carbimazole is the drug of choice it may be ordered in doses of 10 to 20 mg three times daily for a few weeks until the patients symptoms show a satisfactory response. Future control is achieved by maintenance doses of 5 to 15 mg daily.

On occasions Carbimazole is not well tolerated by the patient, in which case Methyl Thiouracil is ordered. Digoxin will be required if atrial fibrillation is present and it is usual for some form of sedation to be given.

Nursing care

Not all patients with thyrotoxicosis are admitted but when required, a bed in a quiet part of the ward is selected in order that initially the patient will not be disturbed by other peoples conditions. The bed clothes will be just enough to cover the patient remembering that these people sweat a lot and also feel the heat somewhat excessively.

Routine temperature, pulse and respirations are taken at four hourly intervals initially with particular reference to the pulse which is also taken when the patient is asleep. Should the nurse detect any irregularities of the pulse then she should also take the apex beat as in all cases of atrial fibrillation.

Diet

As the patients metabolic rate is high, a diet with adequate calorific value should be given together with as much fluid as the patient prefers.

The patients are also grateful for their daily bath and frequent washes due to the excessive sweating. The pressure areas will require frequent attention especially if the patient has lost weight.

Side effect of drugs

Because the antithyroid drugs can produce side effects the nurse should also report if the patient has a sore throat as this may indicate that agranulocytosis has occurred. The physician, when the reduction in the white blood cell count has been confirmed, may stop the treatment. The nurse should also note the presence of skin rashes, nausea, vomiting, diarrhoea and jaundice. She may also notice that the thyroid has increased in size, a fact that may be of interest to the doctor. These patients can be irritable and make demands on nursing time but a calm reassuring approach will eventually be of benefit.

Myxoedema

Clinical features

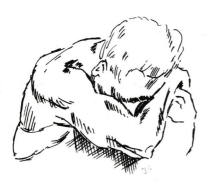

1. Feel cold easily
2. Gains weight
3. Slow mental activity
4. Slow speech
5. Dry skin
6. Hair losses
7. Constipation
8. Tiredness
9. Slow pulse

Treatment

Thyroxine in **gradually** increasing doses

18 Myxoedema

Hypothyroidism or myxoedema is the diagnosis usually applied to patients who present with decreased thyroid function i.e. a lack of thyroxine, but can occasionally arise as a result of thyroidectomy. As with thyrotoxicosis the condition is more common in women and may occur around the time of the menopause, but the onset is variable and may present in earlier life.

Clinical features

The onset is gradual, the features of the disease being due to a lowered metabolism resulting from the deficiency of thyroxine.

The patient may complain that she feels the cold more readily and have noticed a weight gain despite the appetite being poor. Other symptoms include loss of hair, dry skin, an unexplained feeling of tiredness, constipation and hoarseness of the voice.

The skin appears pale and thickened, the face takes on a swollen appearance with the lips being somewhat thicker than normal. The patient does not sweat and the patients relatives may indicate that there has been a slowing down of mental activity and that the speech is slow and monotonous.

The examining physician will find that the pulse is slow together with some enlargement of the heart, with the blood pressure being on the low side. Blood examination reveals a degree of anaemia plus other abnormalities. He will fully investigate the patient in order to exclude other possible diagnoses e.g. Simmonds disease.

Investigations with such tests as radioactive iodine and serum bound protein will indicate that the thyroid concentrates very little iodine and thus tends to aid the diagnosis.

Treatment

The administration of thyroxine is ordered in gradually increasing doses the usual amount being 0.1 mg daily. When the optimum dose has been established the patient continues with the treatment indefinitely. When fully controlled there is a striking difference in the patient who must be warned that the treatment should not be discontinued at any time.

Diabetes mellitus

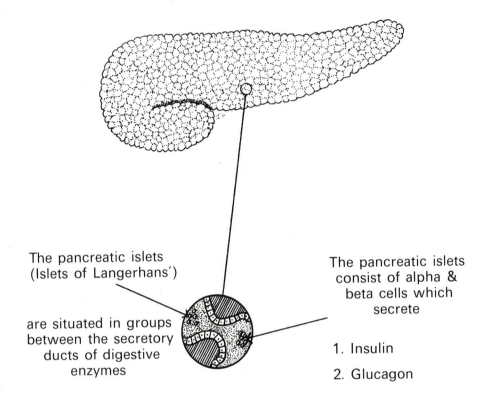

The pancreatic islets
(Islets of Langerhans')

are situated in groups
between the secretory
ducts of digestive
enzymes

The pancreatic islets
consist of alpha &
beta cells which
secrete

1. Insulin

2. Glucagon

Contributing factors

1. Heredity   2. Obesity & overeating

3. Infections   4. Physical & mental stress

5. Endocrine disturbances
e.g. administration of steroids
pancreatectomy

19 Diabetes mellitus

Diabetes mellitus is primarily a condition affecting the metabolism of carbohydrates but also in part that of proteins, fats, water and electrolytes. The condition is extremely common, can occur at any age but the majority of newly diagnosed cases appear after the age of fifty years. The exact aetiology of the condition is unknown but there are several factors which are thought to contribute to the disease. Amongst these factors would be:

1 Familial tendency, in which genetic factors would be involved.
2 Infections which may result in diabetes being diagnosed in its clinical form.
3 Overeating and obesity.
4 Arise as a result of stress in the form of physical injury or emotional disturbance in people who have a latent form of the disease.
5 Arise as a result of pancreatectomy or the administration of corticosteroids.

The disease is one in which hyperglycaemia exists due to the absence or diminution of insulin from the pancreas.

It will be recalled that the Islets of Langerhans in the pancreas make up 1–2% of pancreatic tissue. The cells concerned are named alpha and beta cells, the alpha cells secreting glucagon and the beta cells secreting insulin.

Insulin is required for the conversion of soluble glucose into glycogen in the muscles and liver, and also probably to facilitate the uptake of glucose by the cells of the body.

Glucagon apparently promotes the breakdown of glycogen into glucose and so raises the level of blood sugar, and also probably plays a part in the utilisation of glucose by the tissues. A reduction, or absence of insulin consequently leads to a rise in blood sugar (hyperglycaemia) mentioned above, with particular effect on the individuals carbohydrate metabolism.

Classification of Diabetes

Diabetes can be classified into a number of varying types, but the differences in the clinical picture is one of degree rather than different forms of the disease i.e. they are all diabetic patients. Some authorities divide the condition into two main types:

1 Juvenile onset when occurring in the first forty years of life.
2 Adult maturity onset occurring after forty years.

Nurses will probably be more familar with the classification as follows

1 Severe diabetes which usually applies to childhood and young individuals but it must be remembered that a severe form of the disease can occur at any age.

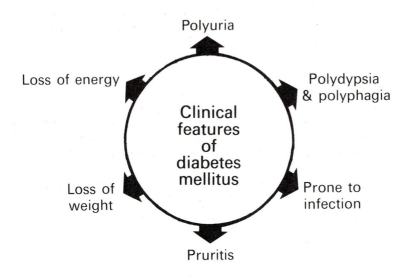

Polyuria

Loss of energy

Polydypsia
& polyphagia

Clinical
features
of
diabetes
mellitus

Loss of
weight

Prone to
infection

Pruritis

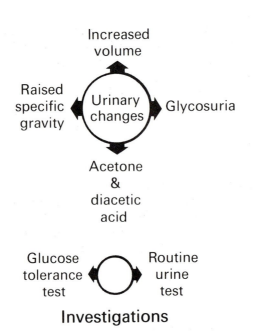

Increased
volume

Raised
specific
gravity

Urinary
changes

Glycosuria

Acetone
&
diacetic
acid

Glucose
tolerance
test

Routine
urine
test

Investigations

2 Moderate diabetes whereby the symptoms are not so severe e.g. the urine is usually free of acetone.
  3 Mild diabetes in which the patient is obese. Again there will be an absence of acetone in the urine but such features as pruritis and polyuria may exist.

Clinical features
  1 Excessive urinary output (polyuria).
  2 Excessive intake of fluids (polydypsia).
  3 Loss of weight despite the appetite being good. The feeling of hunger (polyphagia) is not satisfied with food.
  4 Loss of energy, sometimes accompanied by a feeling of drowsiness.
  5 Pruritis. Itching of the vulva in women and balanitis and inflammation of the glans penis in men.
  6 May be prone to infections such as boils and carbuncles.

Urinary changes
  1 Increased volume.
  2 Raised specific gravity (1,025–1,040).
  3 Glycosuria.
  4 Acetone and diacetic acid may be present.

Hyperglycaemia
The blood sugar level is raised above the normal fasting blood sugar. The normal blood sugar level is about 3.5 mmol/l but rises to about 6 to 6.5 mmol/l after a meal. In diabetes the level rises appreciably higher e.g. 10 mmol/l or more.

It will be recalled that not all diabetic patients will present with the above features. Some mild diabetics may be symptomless, the glycosuria being discovered in some other routine examination.

Investigations
  1 Glucose tolerance test.
    In this test the patient will fast overnight and an oral dose of 50–100 gms of glucose is given. Blood sugar levels are taken before the test and at half hourly intervals up to $2\frac{1}{2}$ hours. A blood glucose level of 10 mmol/l or more is indicative of diabetes.
  2 Routine urine tests.

Treatment
The aims of the treatment are to correct the hyperglycaemia and glycosuria but to maintain the appropriate body weight of the patient. Additionally the diet and insulin control should prevent the onset of hypoglycaemia and try to prevent the onset of complications.

Diabetics, depending upon the type, will be treated by three main methods:

Diabetes is controlled by

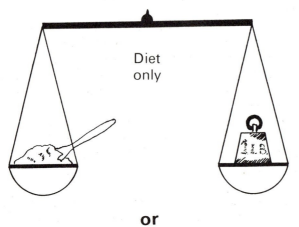

Diet
only

or

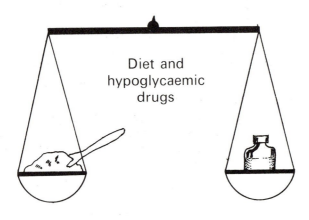

Diet and
hypoglycaemic
drugs

or

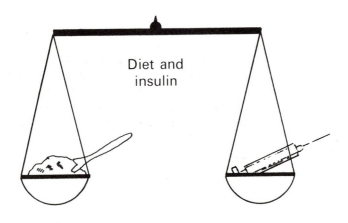

Diet and
insulin

1 Diet alone.
2 Diet and oral hypoglycaemic drugs.
3 Diet and insulin.

It will be noticed that all forms of treatment include dietary control. The diet will take into account the patients age, sex, weight, occupation in order that it is suitable for the individual patients needs. When considering the weight of the patient the physician will take into account the desired weight and not his actual weight.

Most nurses are aware that certain food items can be exchanged for others which will obviously allow for a more varied diet, take into account personal choices, but at the same time keep the total Calorie value of the diet within the limit set by the physician.

Briefly each carbohydrate exchange contains approximately 10 gm of carbohydrate 2 gm of protein and 2/3 gm of fat. Patients will be given lists of exchanges, suggested items for all meals and snacks taken in the day, together with food items which are allowed freely.

Once the diet has been decided upon, the physician will match the insulin or oral hypoglycaemic drug to the carbohydrate content of the diet. An important feature is that painstaking and adequate explanation of the total treatment should be given to the patient.

As indicated earlier care is taken in assessing the energy need of the patient. An approximate range for different groups may be:

1 Young energetic, active patient 2,200–3,000 Calories (8.5–12.5 megajoules).
2 Elderly but not obese patient 1,500–2,200 Calories (6.5–8.5 megajoules).
3 Elderly or obese patient needing to reduce weight 1,200–1,600 Calories (4.75–6.75 megajoules).

Insulin

A variety of different types of insulin are available. Soluble insulin is used initially in order to stabilise new patients who require two injections per day, particularly when the diabetic condition is severe with ketosis present. Many patients have a mixture of soluble insulin and other forms of the preparation e.g. soluble and isophane. When the diabetic control is satisfactory many patients have a once daily injection, e.g. zinc suspension lente. The following table gives the different preparations and their effects:

Preparation	Approximate duration onset	peak	Termination
Soluble	30 minutes	2– 4 hours	6–10 hours
Isophane (NPH)	2–3 hours	4–10 hours	18–24 hours
Globin	2–3 hours	4– 8 hours	10–14 hours

Insulin

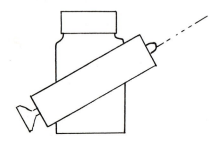

Soluble — Fast acting

Zinc suspension
Semi lente
Lente
P.Z.I.
} Slow acting

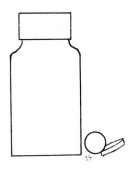

Oral hypoglycaemic agents

Sulphonureas
Biguanides

Nursing care includes:—
Measurement & drawing up of insulin
Sites for injections
Care of syringes & needles
Daily testing of urine

Insulin zinc sus- pension semi lente	2–3 hours	6–10 hours	10–14 hours
Lente (I.Z.S.)	4–6 hours	4–10 hours	18–24 hours
Protamine zinc PZI	4–6 hours	8–10 hours	20–30 hours

Other forms such as Actrapid are also sometimes ordered.

Oral hypoglycaemic drugs

Certain selected patients whose pancreas need a degree of stimulation to produce insulin can be effectively controlled by oral preparations such as Tolbutamide and Chlorpropamide which come under the heading of Sulphonureas; or Phenformin or Metformin which are in a group called Biguanides. The use of these drugs is usually confined to patients in the adult onset group. The doses are between 1–2 gm daily in divided doses for Tolbutamide and Metformin with Chlorpropamide between 100–350 mgms and Phenformin in doses of 50–150 mgms. The drugs are sometimes used in combination.

Nursing care

All new patients being stabilised are taught by the nursing staff how to give the injections and the sites available. They are instructed to vary the site for each injection, the importance of sterility of technique, and also the care of needles and syringes.

As soon as possible patients are also shown how to test their urine and record the colour changes for the presence of glycosuria and acetone.

Other advice given includes the importance of always taking their insulin and to report to their physician when feeling unwell. If they are unable to eat solid food they are advised to look at the list of exchanges in order to take sufficient carbohydrate in another form e.g. glucose or sugar, drinks such as Ribena, Lucozade or Complan. Some patients may also need guidance as to where they can obtain supplies of insulin, syringes and needles but the general practitioner or Health Visitor will be aware of such a need.

Diabetic patients are usually able to lead quite normal lives when they follow the regime as instructed.

Complications of Diabetes Mellitus

Diabetic patients are liable to a number of possible complications, but the main and immediate objective is to keep the patient in employment and free of the troublesome symptoms of the condition. Additionally, the treatment will be aimed at preventing or reducing the risk of more serious complications which can develop despite care by the physician and patient to control the disease.

Complications of diabetes

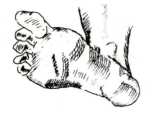 Gangrene of the extremities
due to diminished blood supply

Kidney disease
may develop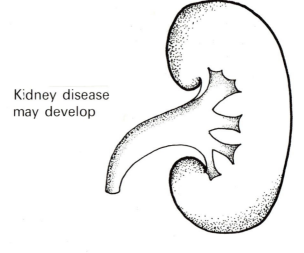

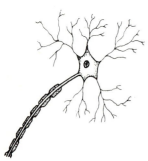 Involvement of the nervous
system — may cause pain or
loss of sensation

Degenerative
lesions may
lead to blindness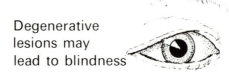

93

The changes which occur in blood vessels account for some of the complications which arise. Thickening of the capillaries develops and results in abnormalities of vision, renal function, and defective circulation. The complications which are of interest to the nurse are as follows.

Diabetic gangrene

Diminished blood supply leading to poorly nourished tissues predisposes to this dangerous complication, particularly if a painless neuropathy (see below) is also present.

Minor injuries to toes perhaps due to careless cutting of toe-nails can be the start of the gangrenous process. All diabetics are advised to have their pedicure carried out by trained chiro-podists. The damaged area is prone to infection and when infected takes a long time to heal.

Elderly diabetics in particular are therefore advised to wear shoes which really fit, avoid hot water bottles in bed as well as taking care not to place their feet too near a hot fire.

When the complication does arise surgery will be necessary. Nurses must always remember the diabetic condition as well as the other post operative measures when nursing patients who have had toes or legs amputated as a result of diabetic gangrene.

Diabetic nephropathy

Patients who have been diabetics for many years can develop kidney disease (Kimmelstiel – Wilson Syndrome) in which there is oedema of the legs, albuminuria, hypertension and uraemia. This complication is often the cause of death in diabetics.

Diabetic neuropathy

The nerves both motor and sensory can be involved, sometimes causing pain in the legs but can also be painless. This means that the patient may ignore or be unaware of some minor injury to the foot or leg and will consequently not seek medical advice.

Diabetic retinopathy

Many patients develop lesions which affect the retina causing a degenerative process. This in turn can lead to blindness due to haemorrhages occurring in the retina.

Infections

Any infection suffered by the patient is of importance particularly in patients who are not well stabilised.

Usually infections such as carbuncles, tonsillitis, pneumonias, renal disease, appendicitis etc. will require an increase in the insulin dosage plus immediate treatment of the infection by antibiotics.

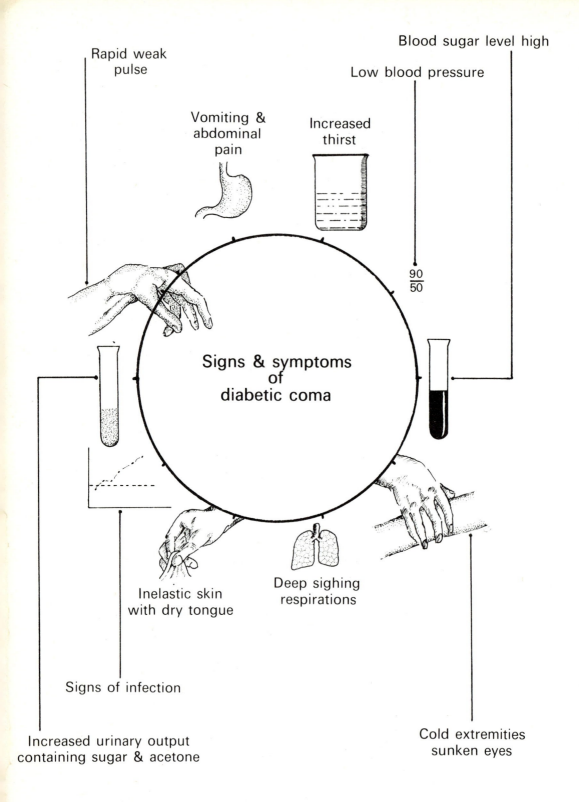

Rapid weak
pulse

Vomiting &
abdominal
pain

Blood sugar level high

Low blood pressure

Increased
thirst

Signs & symptoms
of
diabetic coma

90
50

Inelastic skin
with dry tongue

Deep sighing
respirations

Signs of infection

Increased urinary output
containing sugar & acetone

Cold extremities
sunken eyes

95

Diabetic Coma

The usual cause of diabetic coma in known diabetics is due to the onset of some infection or neglect of the treatment by the patient.

When feeling ill due to infection the patient may not eat the prescribed diet and also omit to take the dose of insulin. As a result the blood sugar rises, ketosis occurs and the patient drifts into coma. Diabetic coma does not happen so frequently nowadays.

The signs and symptoms of diabetic coma are:

1 Onset gradual, the patient will have previously been thirsty, together with an increase in urinary output.
2 Vomiting and abdominal pain.
3 Respirations are deep and sighing with the breath smelling of acetone.
4 Blood pressure is low.
5 Pulse rapid and weak.
6 The skin is inelastic with a dry shrunken tongue.
7 Urine on testing will contain sugar and acetone.
8 Infection is usually present.
9 The extremities feel cold to the touch and the eyeballs give a sunken appearance.
10 Blood sugar level is high.

Treatment

This is a medical emergency and urgent treatment is necessary to restore the patient to consciousness.

The aim is to correct the severe metabolic disorder by treating the ketosis, correct the circulatory collapse by intravenous fluids and to treat the infection by antibiotics.

Insulin: Soluble insulin is given intravenously at first because due to the circulatory collapse absorption via the subcutaneous route is poor. The physician will decide upon the dose to follow the initial intravenous amount which will be given subcutaneously.

IV therapy: An intravenous normal saline drip is set up, the first litre being run through rapidly i.e. within the first hour in order to overcome the dehydration. Later amounts are given at a slower rate.

Urine tests: The patient is catheterised and the urine tested frequently for sugar and acetone. The nurse will be careful in testing because as long as acetone is present the patient is still in danger.

Blood sugar: Blood is taken immediately for blood sugar estimation. When this is very high the physician may increase the dose of insulin to be given.

Further insulin dosage will be determined by the patients progress indicated by blood sugar levels and the degree of ketosis present.

Treatment of diabetic coma

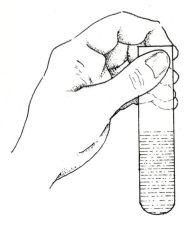

Catheterised urine specimens
frequently tested for:
     sugar
     acetone

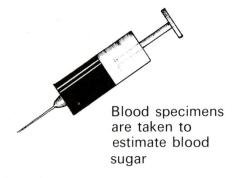

Blood specimens
are taken to
estimate blood
sugar

Intravenous infusions
prevent further
dehydration & correct
circulatory collapse

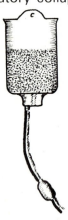

Intravenous soluble
insulin followed
by subcutaneous
doses according
to blood
sugar levels
& urinalysis

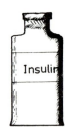

The physician will decide when to give the patient glucose, usually when the sugar content of the urine shows that the amount of sugar is decreasing. Care is taken to avoid any swing from the diabetic coma to a hypoglycaemic attack.

Other nursing measures which can be ordered are gastric lavage and raising the foot of the bed.

As there is a decrease in the potassium level potassium will be given, sometimes orally when the patient has recovered consciousness.

On recovery four hourly feeds of glucose are given usually covered by a suitable dose of insulin.

Any infections present will be treated by antibiotics.

On complete recovery the routine treatment for diabetes is continued and if the patient was an established diabetic then advised further about his condition.

Hypoglycaemia

Some patients who are classified as 'unstable' or 'brittle' diabetics may be prone to severe falls in blood sugar levels. Hypoglycaemia can arise if:

    a More exercise or increased exertion is undertaken.

    b Too much insulin being given.

    c Delayed or irregular meals.

The features of a hypoglycaemic attack are:

1 Onset sudden with feeling of hunger, weakness, palpitation and trembling.
2 Moist skin and tongue.
3 Full pulse with normal or raised blood pressure.
4 Shallow or normal breathing.
5 Urine no acetone.
    no sugar unless the bladder has not been emptied recently.
6 Blood, low blood sugar.

It is possible for the nurse to recognise some of the above signs and take corrective action by giving the patient a glucose drink or if not possible by naso gastric tube. The doctor will give glucose by the intravenous route.

Patients are advised about the symptoms and should carry either sugar lumps or glucose sweets.

Prompt treatment for hypoglycaemic attacks is just as important as the energetic treatment for diabetic coma because if the patient is in coma for several hours then cerebral damage can occur.

All diabetics carry a card or other means of identification stating that they are diabetics.

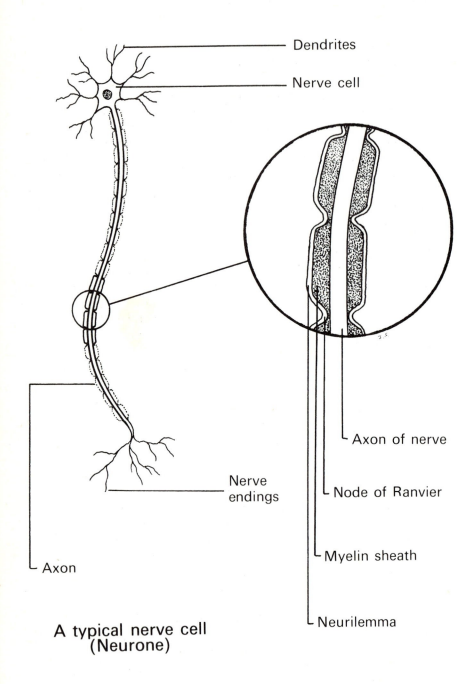

Dendrites

Nerve cell

Axon of nerve

Node of Ranvier

Myelin sheath

Nerve
endings

Neurilemma

Axon

**A typical nerve cell
(Neurone)**

99

20 Diseases of the nervous system

It may be of benefit if before proceeding with specific conditions affecting the nervous system a brief revisionary outline is presented.

The brain and spinal cord are composed of nerve cells (neurones and their processes. The nerve cell constitutes the grey matter of the central nervous system, with the nerve fibres when collected into bundles composing the white matter. The processes are of two kinds and are termed axons and dendrites. The axon conducts impulses *away* from the cell body whilst the dendrite conducts impulses *to* the cell body. Dendrites are usually typically branched (Greek:dendron, a tree) but the axon is always single. The linking of axon to dendrite at the junction of the structures is termed the synapse.

The brain consists of the cerebrum, midbrain, pons, medulla oblongata and the cerebellum. The cerebrum is incompletely divided into two hemispheres each hemisphere being composed of a layer of grey matter, the cerebral cortex, and a deeper mass of nerve fibres called the white matter. The white matter consists of tracts of nerve fibres descending from the cortex and similar tracts ascending to the cortex.

It will be recalled that each cerebral hemisphere is divided into four lobes:

Frontal lobe. Parietal lobe. Temporal lobe. Occipital lobe Each with its own localisation of function (see diagram for detail).

The motor area of the brain is a section of the cortex which lies in front of the fissure of Rolando. This area contains the pyramidal cells the axons of which descend through the internal capsule, midbrain, pons and medulla. These axons connect with the anterior horn cells of the spinal cord and with nuclei in the brain. These nerve fibres transmit impulses governing *voluntary* movements of the body. The motor pathways of the brain and spinal cord (pyramidal tract) consist of fibres from a rather large part of the motor area of the cortex. These tracts cross over in the medulla so that lesions of the right side of the brain will affect the left side of the body and vice versa.

In cerebro vascular accidents the damage may be wide spread as happens when bleeding occurs in the internal capsule, an area in the brain where a large number of nerve fibres pass to and from the brain. As these tracts are motor and sensory there is extensive damage to the conducting pathways, paralysis and often sensory loss occurs (hemiplegia). The offending arteries are branches of the middle cerebral artery. It is also worthwhile remembering that isolated lesions may occur which will result in loss of voluntary movement on a much reduced scale e.g. loss of movement of one limb.

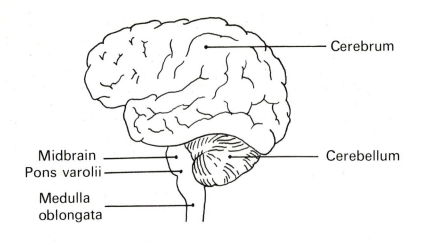

Cerebrum

Midbrain
Pons varolii
Medulla
oblongata

Cerebellum

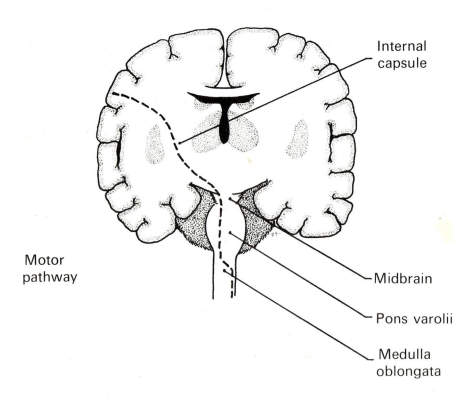

Internal
capsule

Motor
pathway

Midbrain

Pons varolii

Medulla
oblongata

It may be worth recalling that lesions which occur between the cerebral cortex and the anterior horn cell of the spinal cord are termed upper motor neurone lesions. The muscles themselves are not paralysed, the paralysis is of voluntary movement and is spastic. In lower motor neurone disease the lesions affect the anterior horn cells and their processes. Here the muscles are paralysed, the paralysis is flaccid and muscular atrophy follows. The following table gives the major differences between upper motor neurone and lower motor neurone disease.

Upper Motor Neurone	*Lower Motor Neurone*
1 Paralysis or weakness of muscular movement of part of one side of the body.	Weakness or paralysis of muscles.
2 Spastic paralysis. Increased muscle tone and resistance on passive movement.	Flaccid paralysis. i.e. loss of tone on passive movement.
3 Loss of abdominal reflexes.	
4 Tendon reflexes more brisk.	Reflexes absent in area supplied by affected neurone.
5 No muscle wasting.	Muscles subject to contractures.

When examining and investigating the nervous system the physician will assess the motor-sensory and reflex aspects of neurological disorder. He will test for signs of both upper and lower motor neurone lesions together with lesions which may affect the cranial nerves.

Spasticity, power, skin, and other reflexes will be noted. Sensory disturbances of pain, temperature (heat/cold) sense of position, sight, touch, hearing and gait plus others will be looked for. Most nurses are familiar with the tests by which some of the above are elicited.

The reflexes

Mention is made above of the reflexes. These are usually divided into:

Deep tendon reflexes. Superficial reflexes.

The deep tendon reflexes usually examined are:

    1. Knee jerk.   2 Ankle jerk.   3 Arm jerk.

The important point about the deep tendon reflexes is that the pathway used is directed through the lower motor neurone and consequently does not use the pathway of the upper motor neurone. Absence of the deep tendon reflex therefore occurs in diseases of the lower motor neurone. The reflex pathway of the knee jerk is illustrated on page 103.

The superficial reflexes on the other hand use the upper motor pathway and are important investigations in neurological disease. Perhaps the two most likely to be observed by the nurse when she accompanies the physician examining a patient are:

    1 Abdominal reflex.   2 Plantar reflex.

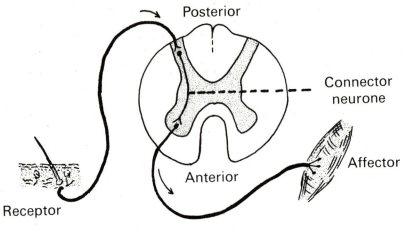

Posterior

Connector
neurone

Affector

Receptor

Anterior

Spinal reflex

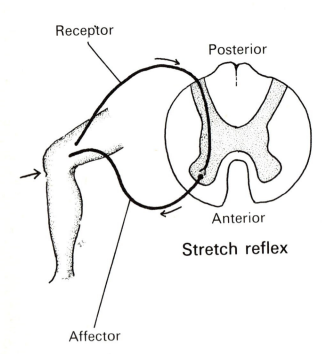

Receptor

Posterior

Affector

Anterior

Stretch reflex

Loss of the abdominal reflex and an altered plantar reflex indicates disease affecting the upper motor neurone. The normal plantar response is for the big toe to turn downwards (flexor response) but disease of the upper motor neurone pathway is indicated by an upward turn of the big toe — Babinski's sign.

Sensory system

Amongst the abnormal features which would be noted when the sensory system is involved would be.

1 Anaesthesia which implies loss of sensation to touch.
2 Hyperaesthesia when there is an increased sensation of touch, indicated by a sensation of tenderness.
3 Paraesthesia when the patient states he has a feeling of 'pins and needles' in the affected area.
4 Analgesia which is a loss of sensation to pain.

   When any of the above occur they usually indicate that the lesion affects the peripheral nerves and do not usually affect the brain.

Thrombosis   Embolism   Haemorrhage

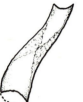 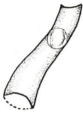 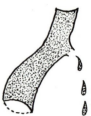

Cerebro vascular accident

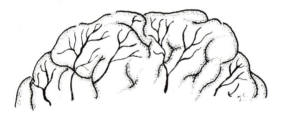

Occurs in the middle meningeal
artery adjacent to the internal capsule

Causes include:—

Atherosclerosis
Sub acute bacterial endocarditis
Mitral stenosis
Coronary thrombosis
Hypertension

21 Cerebro vascular accident

The nurse will come into contact with a number of conditions which are intracerebral in origin but perhaps the most common will be that of stroke or apoplexy. The three more frequently encountered conditions are:

1 Cerebral thrombosis.
2 Cerebral embolism.
3 Cerebral haemorrhage.

Cerebral thrombosis is frequently due to atherosclerosis of a cerebral artery. Cerebral embolism can arise as a result of heart disease such as sub acute bacterial endocarditis, mitral stenosis when atrial fibrillation is present and *coronary thrombosis*. The usual pattern is for a clot to form in the left side of the heart and be carried in the circulation to the brain. The clot will lodge and consequently block one of the cerebral arteries. Cerebral haemorrhage as a cause is often due to an underlying hypertension. It has been previously stated on page 100 that the offending blood vessel is a branch of the middle cerebral arteries i.e. the middle meningeal artery in close relationship with the internal capsule. This blood vessel is very prone to rupture or blockage by a thrombus or embolus.

There is great similarity in the signs and symptoms of all three, the notable difference being in the onset. In both cerebral haemorrhage and embolism the onset is somewhat sudden. Cerebral thrombosis may take a few days to build up before the catastrophe occurs. This cause may present itself when the patient becomes paralysed but not initially become unconscious, but he will probably lapse into coma later.

When the bleed or other cause occurs in the internal capsule the patient usually becomes suddenly unconscious, and if he recovers will be hemiplegic and if the catastrophe has occurred in the left side of the brain, he may also suffer some disorder of speech.

During the unconscious stage the patient is frequently incontinent of both faeces and urine, a feature of obvious nursing significance. It will also be noted that the breathing is deep and rather noisy (stertorous).

The degree of recovery is rather variable. Some patients recover to a remarkable degree whilst in others there is only a minimum power of movement afterwards. The helpful, cheerful, optimistic nurse can be of some comfort to the more severely disabled.

Nursing care
The importance of a clear airway in all stages of unconsciousness is obvious. The patient is usually put in to the semiprone or exaggerated lateral position, naturally the patients position is frequently

Nursing care of
cerebro vascular accident

Clear airway

Correct position
Frequent changes of position

Keep patient dry

Change bedclothes when necessary
Care of skin
Indwelling catheter
Catheter toilet

Oral   toilet

Regular mouth care

Position when conscious

Bed cradles to support bedclothes
Limbs in optimum position
Sandbags to maintain limb position

Physiotherapy
Ambulation
Encouragement

changed in order to prevent both pressure sores and hypostatic pneumonia developing.

Efforts to keep the patient in a dry bed will, together with the above, do much to prevent the onset of pressure sores.

When urinary incontinence is troublesome an indwelling catheter attached to a drainage bag plus regular catheter toilet is probably the best way of caring for this aspect of patient care. Oral toilet is also an obvious part of nursing care.

As indicated earlier a right sided hemiplegia could also result in speech difficulty and the nurse will try to be present when the patient recovers consciousness as he will require quite a degree of support at this time. All efforts should be made to try and really understand the patients needs.

Bed cradles are placed over the patients legs and regular positioning in the optimum position is important, the use of sandbags to maintain the position will be required and must be replaced following a bedbath. Pressure will be avoided on heels which can be kept free of by a judiciously placed small pillow. Other pillows can be placed in strategic positions, depending upon the position in bed. As the paralysis is spastic a small roller bandage or roll of cotton wool placed in the palm of the hand will prevent undue flexion of the fingers. Early ambulation is attempted and encouraged. Physiotherapy of the limbs which are usually put through a full range of passive movements daily, will do much to prevent a bed ridden future existence.

Disseminated sclerosis

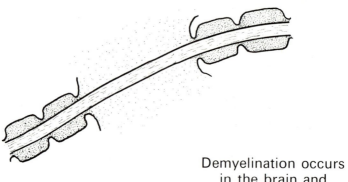

Demyelination occurs
in the brain and
spinal cord

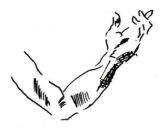

Partial paralysis of a limb
which may recover

Double vision
& nystagmus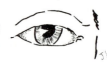

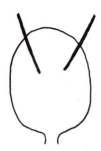

Difficulty of micturition
Incontinence
Retention

22 Multiple sclerosis (Disseminated sclerosis)

This condition is one which comes under the heading of a demyelinating disease, i.e. one in which there are lesions involving the myelin sheath of many neurones.

The cause is unknown but it is thought that in certain cases, genetic factors may be involved.

Pathology

Patches of demyelination occur in a somewhat widespread pattern throughout the brain and spinal cord causing a variety of symptoms. The acute lesion is one in which there is an area where the myelin sheath has undergone destruction and in which irregular swellings of the axis cylinder arise. The lesions are widely scattered in the brain and spinal cord and often involve the optic nerves.

Clinical features

Characteristically the disease runs a course in which following the initial attack, there are remissions and relapses. The relapses may be attributed to, or precipitated by, trauma, infections, or perhaps unusual fatigue.

The widespread lesions result in multiple symptomatology and obviously the site of the plaque will give rise to the particular clinical features.

Age group: The patients are between 20–50 years of age but the incidence is greater in early adult life.

Initially the disease may present itself in the form of partial paralysis of a limb which may last for a short time and clear up. In other patients the presenting symptom may be a visual disturbance in the form of double vision or dimness of vision as a result of retrobulbar neuritis. On occasions the patient may also complain of pain on movement of the eyeball; nystagmus is frequently seen.

Other symptoms include disturbance of bladder function in the form of difficulty in micturition. Incontinence or retention can also be troublesome. There is often a marked tremor which appears on movement and not at rest, consequently termed intention tremor. As the condition progresses speech is also affected whereby there is a peculiar staccato voice (scanning speech).

The disease tends to run a characteristic course in which there are prolonged remissions particularly in the early stages. Young people will present with a variable pattern in which perhaps there will be a transient paralysis of a muscle or group

Paralysis

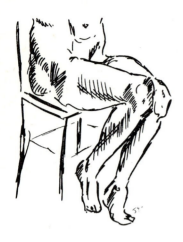

Periods of remission
become less — ataxia
is more pronounced.
Restricted to a wheelchair
and finally bedridden.

Infections are treated
with the appropriate
drug.
A.C.T.H. may be given.

Physiotherapy & occupational therapy
are important.

Basic nursing care is required on
admission to hospital.

of muscles. The other early features of the disease involving vision, or the bladder may or may not be present.

As the disease is a progressive one the periods of remission become less frequent, the paralysis usually of both limbs and the ataxic gait become obvious. Eventually walking even with the aid of sticks becomes impossible and the unfortunate patient is restricted to a wheel chair existence which is later followed by being bedridden and incontinent.

Treatment
There is no specific treatment but during a relapse the patient is nursed in bed, but it is important that the rest period is not prolonged in the early stages. Attempts are made to strike a balance between too much activity and too much rest, the patient must not be overfatigued.

Infections particularly urinary infections are treated accordingly. An injection of ACTH may be given.

Physiotherapy together with occupational therapy are important forms of treatment.

Nursing care
When admitted to hospital the patient will require all the basic nursing care of bedbaths, pressure area care, attention to diet and of course particular care with incontinence of urine. Enemata for constipation may also be required.

Some patients appear to be euphoric and the nurse must also present an attitude of reasoned optimism and hope, particularly when the patient is relatively young.

The cranial nerves

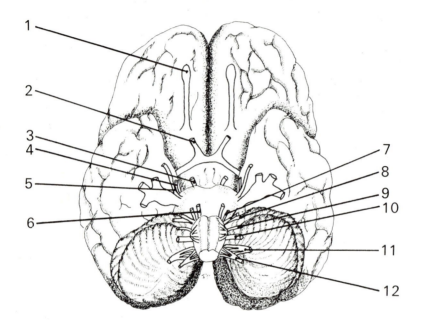

1. Olfactory
2. Optic
3. Oculomotor
4. Trochlear
5. Trigeminal
6. Abducent

7. Facial
8. Auditory
9. Glossopharyngeal
10. Vagus
11. Accessory
12. Hypoglossal

23 The cranial nerves

When discussing diseases of the nervous system, mention is often made of the cranial nerves due to their involvement in such conditions. The nerves, together with certain specific conditions which could affect them will be taken in consecutive order and discussed briefly.

1 The olfactory nerve arises from the receptors situated in the nasal mucosa, pass through the cribriform plate of the anterior fossa of the skull to the brain and finally synapse in the olfactory bulb and thence to the olfactory area in the frontal lobe.

The only point of interest to the nurse is that tumours of the frontal lobe can cause loss of smell and that damage to the nerves can arise as a result of head injuries.

2 The optic nerve. Visual impulses from the retina pass back via the optic nerve to the occipital area of the brain. The more exact details of the visual pathways is shown on page 115 which shows the pathway taken by the temporal and nasal fibres. Examination of the eye is an extremely important investigation in diseases of the central nervous system and other conditions.

Papilloedema: on examination of the retina by means of the ophthalmoscope, the physician can see the swelling of the optic disc. Conditions which give rise to papilloedema include:

  a diseases of the retinal arteries which occur in malignant hypertension.
  b increased intracranial pressure e.g. in meningitis or cerebral tumour.

Optic neuritis: This can be due to, or as a manifestation of disseminated sclerosis. There are other causes but perhaps the above will be more familiar to most nurses due to the demyelination of the nerves involved.

Optic atrophy: Can arise from a large number of causes amongst which would be glaucoma and diabetes mellitis.

3 The occulomotor nerve supplies all extrinsic muscles of the eye except the superior oblique and the lateral rectus. It is also the constrictor supply to the pupil and the ciliary muscle as well as supplying the upper eye lid.

Conditions which can arise from lesions of the third cranial nerve include strabismus and drooping of the eye lid (ptosis). The nerve can also be affected in diabetes mellitis, disseminated sclerosis and other diseases. As the nerve is constrictor to the pupil paralysis of the nerve will result in dilation of the pupil.

4 The trochlear nerve supplies the superior oblique muscle of the eye consequently damage to the nerve will affect the movement of the eyeball.

5 The trigeminal nerve is both motor and sensory and supplies by its three branches the ophthalmic, mandibular and maxillary

The visual pathways

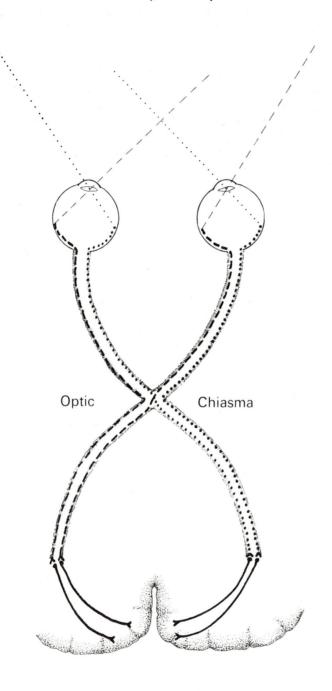

Optic   Chiasma

areas of the face, the cornea, mucous membrane of the nose, the teeth and part of the tongue. Perhaps the two most familiar conditions affecting the nerve are shingles (herpes zoster) and trigeminal neuralgia.

6 The abducent nerve supplies the lateral rectus of the eyeball. Any lesion which affects this nerve will, similar to the nerves of other muscles of the eyeball, cause strabismus and diplopia.

7 The facial nerve supplies the muscles of facial expression and also the taste buds in the anterior part of the tongue. Bell's palsy is a condition which occurs in lesions of this nerve. The nerve also passes through the middle ear, consequently it can be damaged by inflammatory processes within the middle ear. Cerebral haemorrhage involving the internal capsule can also affect the nerve and may perhaps be the involvement most frequently seen by the nurse.

8 The auditory nerve. This nerve has two components, the cochlear branch which is concerned with hearing and the vestibular branch which is concerned with appreciation of the movement of the head in space.

Cochlear lesions: conduction deafness can result from inflammatory middle ear diseases.

Vestibular lesions: cause vertigos and imbalance, a condition which may be encountered by the nurse in Meniere's syndrome in which there is a combination of tinnitus, deafness and vertigo.

Tinnitus may be an early symptom of an acoustic neuroma. Most nurses will recall that the eighth cranial nerve can be damaged by the toxic effects of dihydrostreptomycin and that damage can also be caused by meningitis.

The remaining nerves ninth, tenth, eleventh and twelfth all leave the medulla and are in such close proximity that any lesion is likely to affect all four. There are no conditions of particular nursing interest.

Epilepsy

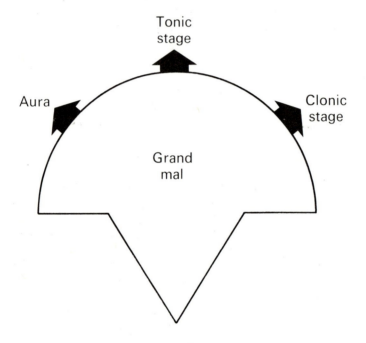

Tonic
stage

Aura

Clonic
stage

Grand
mal

Diagnosis

History
Examination of the nervous system
Electroencephalogram
Skull Xray
Urinalysis, blood pressure
Laboratory examination of blood

      I. Urea
     II. Wasserman test
    III. Kahn test

24 Epilepsy

An epileptic fit is a condition in which there is a sudden and excessive electrical discharge of cerebral neurones causing a brief disorder of cerebral function and loss of consciousness.

The aetiology is somewhat obscure, but heredity appears to play a part. Predisposing factors include such causes as birth injuries, neoplastic lesions, vascular lesions and trauma of the brain. The major form of epilepsy, grand mal, will be considered in detail.

Grand mal

This fit usually presents in a particular clinical pattern in which the nurse can recognise many stages.

1　There may have been a change of mood lasting for hours or days.

2　*Aura* usually of very brief duration which can take many forms.

3　The *tonic stage* occurring at onset. The patient loses consciousness and falls to the ground. The muscles are in a state of sustained tonic spasm, which also involves the respiratory muscles. Air passing through the partially closed glottis gives rise to the epileptic cry. Cyanosis occurs because respiratory movements are suspended, the duration being about 20–30 seconds.

4　The *clonic stage* lasts about 30–40 seconds, during which the muscles are seen to produce powerful jerky movements of limbs, body and face. The tongue and jaw move and the patient froths at the mouth. Incontinence can occur at this stage.

5　When the clonic stage ceases the patient becomes flaccid, comatose, and usually proceeds to a normal sleep lasting from minutes to hours. The patient on recovering consciousness usually complains of a severe headache. Some patients may proceed into a post epileptic automatism in which they become antisocial and may involuntarily commit criminal acts.

Diagnosis

As there are different forms of epilepsy, the doctor will be interested in the nature of the attack. Epilepsy is a symptom and the investigations will perhaps help to discover why the fits occurred.

Besides a full examination of the nervous system plus taking a history of any familial tendency, it is probable that an EEG (electroencephalogram) will be ordered together with a skull X ray. Routine measures include urine tests, blood pressure, blood urea examination and a Wasserman reaction and Kahn

Treatment

Protect the patient from injury.
Loosen tight clothing at neck & waist
Prevent tongue being bitten

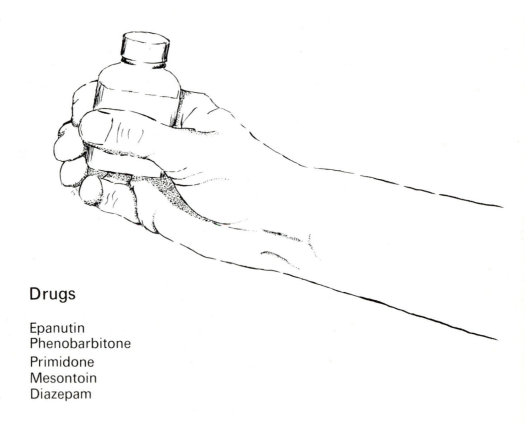

Drugs

Epanutin
Phenobarbitone
Primidone
Mesontoin
Diazepam

test, the last two being performed in order to exclude any suggestion of cerebral syphilis.

Treatment

During a fit one of the main duties is to prevent the patient injuring himself consequently all movable furniture is moved a short distance from the patient or if necessary move the patient from the danger.

Any tight clothing is loosened especially about the neck and waist. No undue restraint should be used in the clonic stage but arm and leg movements can be directed if required in order to prevent any further damage.

The preventative treatment instituted is aimed at an amelioration of the effects of fits by reducing their frequency. Drugs used include phenobarbitone 60—90 mgs three times daily but this may be varied according to the patients age and possibly the severity of the fits.

Epanutin (phenytoin sodium) can also be prescribed 100 mgs three times daily. Other anticonvulsive preparations which may be ordered include Primidone, Mesontoin and Diazepam. As some of the drugs cause toxic effects, care and control will be required, e.g. anaemia may occur as a result of the treatment.

Social factors

Adults suffering from epilepsy will find certain jobs barred to them. Obviously, work involving machinery or climbing scaffolding or ladders could not be considered. Similarly driving vehicles either privately or as a means of employment *should also be avoided*. Many well controlled epileptics however do hold responsible jobs. It should be the aim that all epileptics lead as normal a life as possible. Children will need to continue education without too much restriction placed on their activities.

Status Epilepticus

In this condition fits will follow each other in rapid succession and can continue for many hours. Urgent treatment in hospital is required as this is a very dangerous condition which can lead to death from exhaustion. Treatment will be directed to:

1 Maintenance of an adequate airway.
2 Suppression of the fits.

Drugs are given intramuscularly or on occasions intravenously when the attack is of a very severe nature.

Sodium phenobarbitone 200 mgs will be ordered or Phenytoin in 250 mg doses may be prescribed. Paraldehyde is frequently ordered to be given in doses of 10 mls with smaller doses being given at half hourly intervals. Diazepam may also be given intravenously but is given slowly in doses of 10 mgs. Another preparation which is sometimes used intravenously is Thiopentone.

Status epilepticus

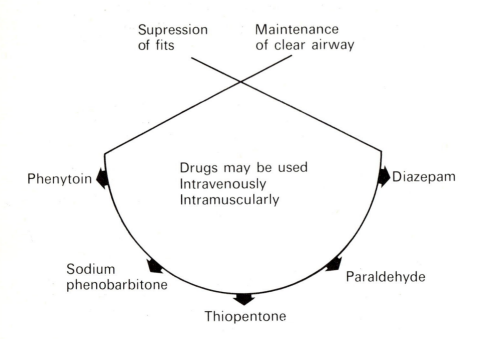

Supression
of fits

Maintenance
of clear airway

Phenytoin

Drugs may be used
Intravenously
Intramuscularly

Diazepam

Sodium
phenobarbitone

Paraldehyde

Thiopentone

Other forms of epilepsy

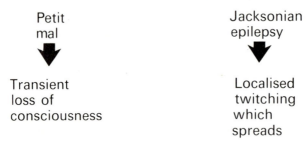

Petit
mal

Jacksonian
epilepsy

Transient
loss of
consciousness

Localised
twitching
which
spreads

It can be somewhat distressing to care for a patient in status epilepticus but if at all possible the nurse should try to keep a record of the number of fits. Efforts to prevent the patient injuring himself will be required but it will be noted that usually there is no incontinence in status epilepticus. It will also be noted that frequently the patient is hyperpyrexial, the hyperpyrexia plus the exhaustion of prolonged attacks can lead to a fatal outcome.

Petit mal

Nurses may have contact with this condition in patients admitted for other reasons. The individual has a transient loss of consciousness, stares blankly into space, and stops what he was doing or saying. The whole episode lasts for a very brief period of time i.e. 10–15 seconds. Following the attack the patient then resumes his activities.

It is seen mainly in children, can persist into adult life or may cease during adolescence. Sometimes the condition develops into grand mal epilepsy.

Jacksonian epilepsy

In this condition the twitching movements will start in one area of the body and spread to involve other regions. It may start in one limb or part of a limb and spread in a progressive order to involve perhaps the whole body. Consciousness is not always lost and the nurse observing such a fit from the beginning could note the order in which the muscles are involved and report accordingly.

Meningitis

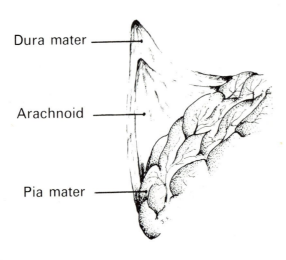

Dura mater

Arachnoid

Pia mater

Causative organisms

Pyogenic meningitis

I. Meningococcus
II. Pneumococcus
III. Haemophilus influenzae
IV. Staphylococcus & streptococcus

Tuberculous meningitis

Viral meningitis

25 Meningitis

Inflammation of the meninges, more specifically the pia mater and arachnoid mater, arises from infection by a number of organisms. The types most commonly encountered are mentioned below.

1 *Pyogenic meningitis* which is caused by a number of pus forming organisms resulting in the following types of meningitis.
  a Meningococcal meningitis also called cerebrospinal fever or spotted fever.
  b Pneumococcal.
  c Influenzal caused by Haemophilus influenzae.
  d Staphylococcal and Streptococcal.
The Meningococcal, Pneumococcal and Influenzal forms of the disease are acute in onset usually resulting in very severe types of infection. The meningococcal form is spread by droplet infection but the pneumococcal and influenzal type is often secondary to infection somewhere else in the body.

The staphylococcal and streptococcal types may arise from infection of the middle ear (otitis media) or due to further spread from mastoiditis or sinusitis.

2 *Tuberculous meningitis.* This condition is spread via the blood stream from a focus somewhere else in the body, but unlike the acute onset of the previously mentioned types, the onset is more gradual.

3 *Viral meningitis.* Not so severe as other forms but appears to be more frequently encountered in recent years.

Clinical features
Whatever the type of infection, the clinical features are the same for all forms being due to the inflammation causing increased meningeal irritation.
  1 Onset is acute with the exception (tuberculous) given above.
  2 Pyrexia which can be high and often associated with rigors.
  3 Headache which rapidly becomes severe and constant. The patient may complain that the headache spreads down the back of the neck.
  4 Vomiting which together with the headache is often significant of increased intracranial pressure.
  5 Photophobia, whereby the patient turns away from the light.
  6 The patient is often confused, resents interference and lies curled up on his side.
  7 Convulsions particularly in children are present at the onset.
  8 Neck rigidity. The patient complains of neck stiffness and any attempt to flex the head is strongly resisted.

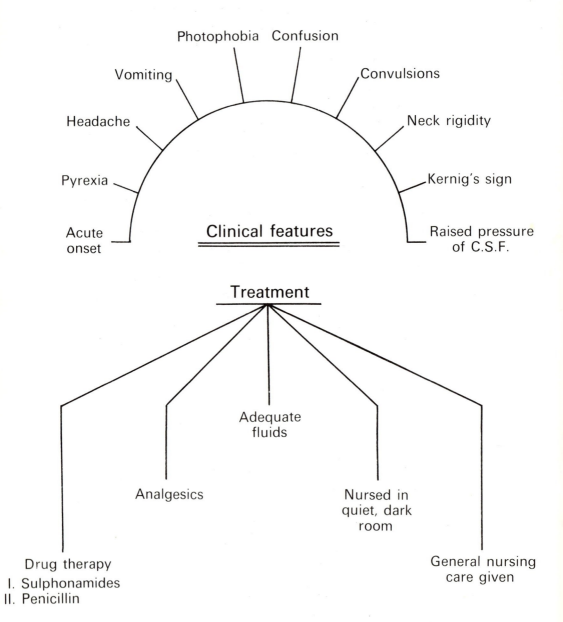

Photophobia Confusion

Vomiting

Convulsions

Headache

Neck rigidity

Pyrexia

Kernig's sign

Acute
onset

Clinical features

Raised pressure
of C.S.F.

Treatment

Adequate
fluids

Analgesics

Nursed in
quiet, dark
room

Drug therapy
I. Sulphonamides
II. Penicillin

General nursing
care given

Kernig's sign. This means that there is resistance when attempts are made to straighten the flexed knee joint due to spasm of the hamstring muscles.

The pain caused by attempts to flex the neck or elicit Kernig's sign, is due to the stretching of the meninges. The patient consequently resists the physicians attempts to place the chin on the chest or to straighten the knee joint with the leg at an angle of 90° to the abdomen.

Diagnosis

In addition to the symptoms and signs in evidence, a lumbar puncture is performed. The CSF will be under pressure and be turbid in appearance due to the large increase in white blood cells, characteristically polymorphonuclear leuocytes.

Treatment

It is customary for drug therapy to be commenced without waiting for any bacteriological confirmation.

Drugs used are Sulphadimidine or Sulphadiazine, the physician ordering a particular course of the drug chosen. Should the need arise, e.g. vomiting, then the drug is given by the intramuscular or intravenous route. On occasions antibiotics such as Penicillin or Tetracycline are used, sometimes in combination with the Sulphonamides.

Analgesics for the relief of pain or headache can also be ordered. In some forms of meningitis penicillin preparations can be given intrathecally.

Nursing care

The patients are best nursed in a quiet area. The room will be warm, well ventilated, and due to the photophobia the lighting will be subdued.

All efforts must be made, despite the irritability of the patient to ensure an adequate fluid intake, flavoured glucose drinks being frequently offered. As with all very ill toxic patients, oral toilet will make the patient feel better and more able to tolerate a light diet once the specific treatment begins to take effect. Care of skin, pressure areas and daily bed baths will also do much for the patients comfort.

Tuberculous meningitis

Tubercular meningitis is always secondary to tuberculous infections in other regions of the body. The onset is insidious.

Lumbar puncture will show a raised pressure and the diagnosis is confirmed by microscopic examination of the CSF for Mycobacterium tuberculosis.

Treatment is by administering the usual drugs used in tuberculosis i.e. Isoniazid, PAS and Streptomycin.

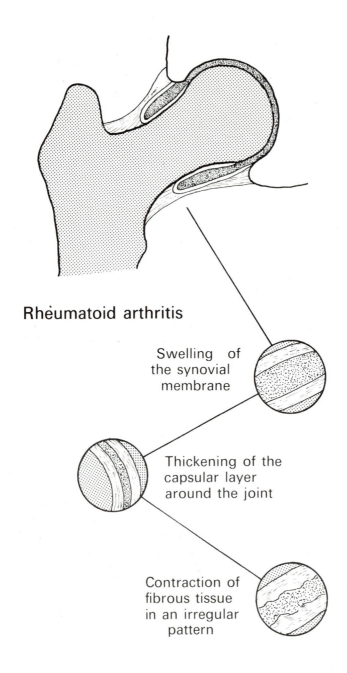

Rheumatoid arthritis

Swelling of
the synovial
membrane

Thickening of the
capsular layer
around the joint

Contraction of
fibrous tissue
in an irregular
pattern

26 Diseases of connective tissue

Rheumatism
Many individuals complain of aches and pains in muscles and joints, some of which are vaguely labelled rheumatism. Such conditions are the cause of much loss of work and account for many millions of pounds to industry. Some rheumatic diseases can result in both temporary and permanent disability.

Rheumatoid arthritis
This condition is relatively widespread and in many instances result in the sufferer being severely disabled or bedridden.

In effect, the disease is one in which there is a swelling of the synovial membrane and the adjacent connective tissue leading later to hypertrophy of the membrane, together with a thickening of the capsular layer around the joint. The fibrous tissue formed contracts in a somewhat irregular fashion which results in an apparent deformity in the joint. Most nurses will have seen the altered positions of alignment in many patients where the individual kept the joint flexed because this position gives ease from the pain. Women are affected more frequently than men, the age of onset being after 40 years but any age can be affected. In children the condition is called Still's disease.

Clinical features
The onset can be insidious in many patients, with the individual complaining of some joint pain and also of a feeling of general tiredness and fatigue. Classically the first joints to be affected are the fingers or toes but the disease can later involve the larger joints such as the wrists, ankles, elbows, shoulders and knees.

The patient will feel a stiffness and pain in the affected joint particularly on rising from bed in the morning, the thickening and pain in the joint causing some reduction in mobility. Sometimes the degree of pain experienced may be severe enough to disturb sleep, this being particularly so as the disease progresses.

There are periods of remission, but during the acute phase the patient will have a low grade pyrexia, a degree of tachycardia plus a degree of anaemia. A blood test will show a raised erythrocyte sedimentation rate.

Treatment
The treatment is aimed towards the relief of the symptoms, a general improvement in the patients health and to prevent if possible further disability; These will be considered under three headings.

1 General.   2 Local.   3 Specific or drug therapy.

Treatment

General

─── Rest

      I. Physical
      II. Mental

─── Firm mattress
or fracture boards

─── High protein diet
      Milk
      Iron for anaemia

─── Controlled physiotherapy

Immobilisation
of painful joints ─── **Local**

Application of heat ───

Occupational therapy ───

Active physiotherapy ───

1 General measures

Rest both physical and mental are very important features particularly during any acute phase. The nurse will see that the bed has a firm mattress or that fracture boards are inserted if a softer mattress is used. A limited number of pillows and a firm backrest are allowed with a bed cradle placed in position over the legs. The care and rest in bed will do much to relieve the symptoms particularly if the joints affected are weight bearing.

In order to maintain mobility, active, but careful physiotherapy is performed daily with the nurse assisting with quadriceps extensor exercises and foot, wrist and hand movements, the above being ordered when the acute phase has subsided.

The diet ordered will have a high protein content, the nurse seeing that the meal is cut up and manageable by the patient if this is required i.e. if the deformity in the hands makes the manipulation of a knife and fork difficult. Iron will probably be ordered in order to correct the anaemia. Flavoured milk drinks are a useful supplement to the patients diet because milk contains first class protein and calcium.

2 Local measures

Painful joints are usually immobilised in light but skin tight plaster of Paris splints, and are usually maintained in position until the acute symptoms have subsided. The splints may well be in position for one to two weeks, and after removal the patient is encouraged to perform any non weight bearing exercises ordered. Local application of heat is beneficial, other forms of heat may be by radiant heat, infra red rays or shortwave diathermy. More active physiotherapy and occupational therapy are also used to restore the patient to a more normal pattern of activity.

3 Drug therapy

The most frequently used drug is *Aspirin* which is both analgesic, and in the doses ordered, anti-inflammatory. Soluble aspirin in doses of 4—6 g in 24 hours is the usual dose. Some physicians order Codeine phosphate tablets (30 mgs) to be given also if the pain is particularly severe.

Other anti-inflammatory drugs used include Indomethacin in doses from 25 mgs to 75 mgs daily. The drug can give rise to nausea, vomiting, headache and dizziness. Phenylbutazone (Butazolidine) which can relieve the pain, in doses of 100 mgs three times a day can also be prescribed, but this drug can give rise to side effects particularly gastric bleeding, blood dyscrasias, rashes and some oedema due to sodium retention. More commonly they cause nausea and vomiting.

A derivative of Butazolidine is a drug called Oxyphenbutazine (Tanderil) and is sometimes employed instead of Butazolidine.

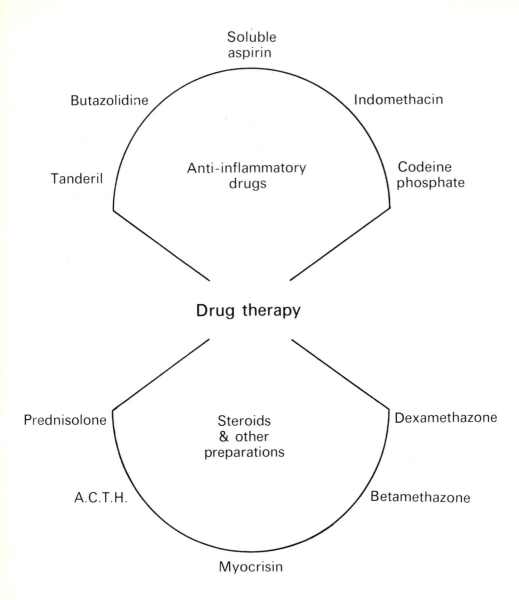

Soluble aspirin

Butazolidine

Indomethacin

Tanderil

Anti-inflammatory drugs

Codeine phosphate

Drug therapy

Prednisolone

Steroids & other preparations

Dexamethazone

A.C.T.H.

Betamethazone

Myocrisin

Steroids

The most frequently employed drugs appear to be Prednisolone, Dexamethazone and Betamethazone. The doses are carefully considered by the physician and are used with due caution.

ACTH (Corticotrophin) which stimulates the patients own adrenals is also used. Other preparations include gold salts (Myocrisin) given in divided doses over a period of weeks until one gramme has been given. Sometimes gold salts are given in conjunction with steroids. When a patient is on a series of gold salt injections the nurse should test the urine for protein, which if present should be reported. The urine is tested *before* the injection is given.

Conclusion

The treatment of rheumatoid arthritis is frequently a team effort involving the physician, physiotherapists and occupational therapists. The orthopaedic surgeon is also often involved in some forms of treatment. In the home situation, the social service workers are of great benefit, being able to offer advice and assistance in coping with both the physical handicaps and the geography of the home.

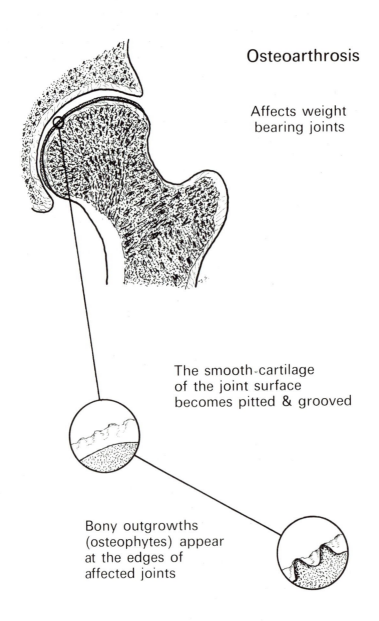

Osteoarthrosis

Affects weight bearing joints

The smooth cartilage of the joint surface becomes pitted & grooved

Bony outgrowths (osteophytes) appear at the edges of affected joints

27 Osteoarthrosis

Osteoarthrosis or osteoarthritis is a degenerative condition of the cartilage which covers the ends of long bones. Normally the cartilage forms a smooth glistening surface which allows free and easy movement of the joint surfaces. In the diseased state, the cartilage loses its hard smooth appearance and becomes pitted and grooved, particularly at the point of maximum weight bearing. Small bony outgrowths called osteophytes appear at the edge of the affected joints. The larger joints such as the hip and knee are most commonly affected, particularly in individuals who are overweight. There may be a history of trauma to the joint some years previously or it can arise in occupations where there has been continual stress on certain joints e.g. coal miners.

Clinical features

Pain is intermittent at first with the symptoms being insidious in onset. The pain appears especially when the joint has been used and following a period of rest. As the condition develops movement in the affected joint becomes increasingly difficult and limited, due to the associated muscle spasm, loss of cartilage and the formation of osteophytes. Examination of the joint will show muscle wasting to a lesser or greater degree.

Diagnosis

X ray of the area will indicate the loss of joint space as well as show up the osteophytes if present.

Treatment

Obese patients will obviously be urged to diet and so lose weight. Pain will be relieved by periods of rest during the day if at all possible. Heat treatment by the physiotherapist, together with some form of gentle exercise will also relieve the pain and stiffness.

Drugs such as Aspirin and Codeine are given, but the physician will consider using Phenylbutazone if the pain is persistent. Other forms of treatment include intra-articular injections of Steroids, hydrotherapy and surgery. It may be necessary in certain cases for a change of occupation to be considered, particularly if the existing occupation is one which places undue stress on the affected joint. The changes which have taken place in the joint are irreversible, consequently the treatment ordered is aimed at relieving the symptoms.

Surgery

Nowadays the advice of the orthopaedic surgeon is sought in the treatment of the condition, particularly when the disability is such as to prevent walking. A variety of operative procedures are considered amongst which are Arthroplasty Arthrodesis or osteotony.

Prurines break down to
uric acid in excessive
amounts

Raising the
level of
uric acid
in the blood

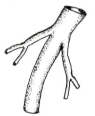

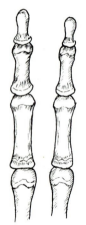

Uric acid
settles in
the joints
and cartilage

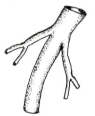

causing **Gout**

28 Gout

This condition arises from a disorder of certain types of protein named prurines present in the nuclei of tissue cells. The nucleo-protein is broken down, finally ending as uric acid, the source being from both exogenous and endogenous protein. Excessive breakdown of these nucleoproteins results in a raised level of uric acid in the blood which settles in the joints and cartilages. It may be worth noticing that patients with myeloid leukaemia can occasionally suffer from gout due to the excessive breakdown of large numbers of leukaemic cells, which in turn raise the levels of uric acid.

The nodules which arise in certain areas of the body e.g. lobes of the ears, fingers, back of the hand etc. are called tophi and consist of deposits of urates which have formed. These can vary in size, the underlying skin is thin and on occasions the tophi can ulcerate and so become infected.

Diagnosis
Confirmation of the condition can be made by extracting from the tophus some of the enclosed material and examining micro-scopically, or by estimating from a blood sample the level of uric acid which will be raised if the disorder is present.

Clinical features
1 Acute arthritic pain is felt in the affected joint, frequently the big toe, but can arise in other joints also.
2 The onset can be sudden, often at night time, the joint becoming swollen, red and extremely painful.
3 The patient is very irritable, restless with a degree of fever.
4 Other features include malaise and leucocytosis.
5 Later there appears some desquamation of the skin followed by some local itching.

Treatment
In the acute episode the physician may order Phenybutazone 100 mgs three times daily or Colchicine 0.5 mg every two hours. Aspirin is often ordered to be given with Colchicine.

The usual care is taken when Phenylbutazone is ordered due to its unplesant toxic effects, which can cause gastric ulcers and agranulocytosis. Obviously, the drug would be avoided as long term therapy. Colchicine may cause diarrhoea in certain patients.

Steroids in the form of Prednisolone may be given, but as is customary the dose of the drug is tailed off once the symptoms are relieved.

Nursing care
The affected joint can be wrapped in warm cotton wool and the affected limb well supported. A bed cradle will keep the weight

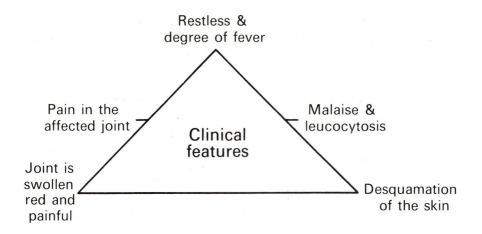

Restless &
degree of fever

Pain in the
affected joint

Malaise &
leucocytosis

Clinical
features

Joint is
swollen
red and
painful

Desquamation
of the skin

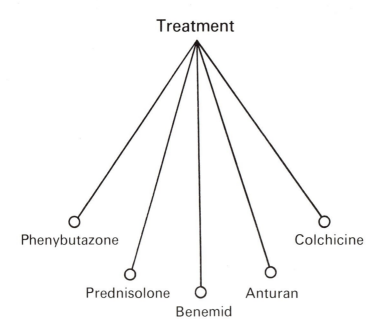

Treatment

Phenybutazone

Colchicine

Prednisolone

Benemid

Anturan

of the bed clothes off the affected area but care must be taken to prevent any injury to the joint. Dressings of lotio plumbi et opii (lead and opium) may also be ordered.

Chronic gout
If overweight a reducing diet is ordered, otherwise the only diet restriction is to avoid food with a high prurine content and also any alcoholic excess. It is advisable for the patients to drink four to five pints of fluid daily which will reduce the chance of urates being deposited in the kidneys.

Drugs which increase the excretion of uric acid from the body are ordered. These drugs act by reducing the reabsorption of uric acid from the renal tubule. Two such drugs are:

1 Anturan (Sulphinpyrazone) 50–100 mgs four times daily.
2 Benemid (Probenecid) 0.5 mg four times daily.

The drugs must be taken for the remainder of the patients life to be effective.

Obesity

Causes:-
1. Genetic
2. Pregnancy
3. Menopause
4. Psychological

May be a predisposing
factor to—

Gall stones
Myocardial infarction
Osteoarthrosis
Gout
Hypertension
Varicose veins

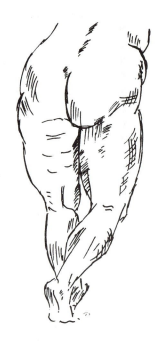

Treatment

Restrict carbohydrate intake
Restrict alcohol
Take exercise
May be prescribe—appetite suppressants

29 Obesity

Basically, obesity is the result of eating more food than the individual requires, the effect of the condition being wide spread in that extra effort is required for all activity and is a hazard to health. Obvious examples of conditions where obesity could be a predisposing cause, include gall stones, myocardial infarction, osteoarthrosis, gout, hypertension, varicose veins and others. Perhaps the motor car which obviously makes people take less exercise i.e. walking, could also be a contributory factor.

The cause of obesity is not always apparent, but can arise after pregnancy and the menopause, there are also genetic factors which may be of influence. Obesity may tend to run in families, but again this may be due to the eating pattern of the family.

Psychological factors also play their part, some women over eat when under emotional stress or are unhappy for some reason or another. There does not appear to be much support amongst doctors that endocrine disturbances are to blame.

Treatment

Diet
Whatever the reason for the obese state, patients will need to be encouraged by the nurse to stick to their diet. Usually the diet has been formulated with a view to severely restricting its carbohydrate content. Sweet foods such as chocolate, sugar, cakes, biscuits etc. are forbidden but the protein content is within normal limits. Fried dishes are best avoided. Although fluids are allowed it is worthwhile reminding the patient that alcoholic drinks particularly beer and stout all add to the number of Calories allowed per day.

In addition to reducing food intake it will be worthwhile reminding the patient that exercise will also reduce weight by expending energy, but this may be difficult if the patient has some accompanying disability.

Anorectic drugs
Nowadays drugs are available which can only aid the patient to keep to their prescribed diets, that is the drugs act as appetite suppressants.

Amongst such drugs are Amphetamine, Dexamphetamine, Fenfluramine and many others. As with all drugs there are dangers in that they can be habit forming. The potentially serious effects of overdose should also be kept in mind and consequently should not be within the reach of children.

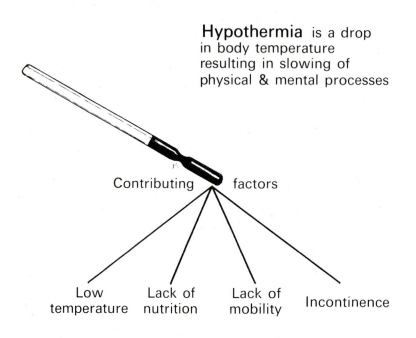

Hypothermia is a drop in body temperature resulting in slowing of physical & mental processes

Contributing factors

Low temperature   Lack of nutrition   Lack of mobility   Incontinence

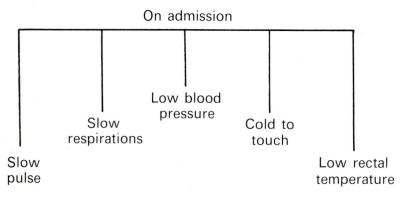

On admission

Slow pulse   Slow respirations   Low blood pressure   Cold to touch   Low rectal temperature

Care is necessary to warm the patient **slowly**

30 Hypothermia

In hypothermia the body temperature drops, causing all the chemical processes of the body to slow down including the mental process which becomes sluggish.

Old people, and sometimes babies lose heat from the body quicker than they can create heat. When the external temperature is very cold, despite what is apparently adequate protection from bedclothes the victim can gradually proceed into a state of hypothermia.

The situation can be made worse by lack of nutrition, incontinence, perhaps lack of mobility due to other diseases e.g. arthritis. On occasions there is sufficient fuel in the home and adequate nutrition is available, but when individuals have reached a certain degree of hypothermia they cannot rouse themselves to get warm possibly due to their sluggish mental state.

These patients become confused, drowsy and can fall asleep in a chair in an already very cold room. Many organs in the body are damaged, with small thrombi forming in blood vessels. If they are not found soon enough they become comatose and die.

On admission the patient will be seen to have slow respirations, very slow pulse and low blood pressure. Rectal temperature is low and the body cold to touch.

The thermometer used must be one which registers low temperatures.

The treatment is obviously to warm the body by warm blankets with constant readings of temperature. Intravenous hydrocortisone can be administered together with some form of antibiotic. The physician will determine any electrolyte imbalance and correct it accordingly. The patients are connected to a monitor or an ECG is taken which will indicate any cardiac irregularities.

The nurse will take particular care with the warming up process, keeping records of temperature, pulse, respirations and blood pressure, taken at regular frequent intervals. When warming up the patient heat must not be applied directly to the skin and the use of heavy blankets, heated cradles, electric blankets and hot water bottles are best avoided. Much will depend on how long the patient has been hypothermic before being found, and if they are going to recover, obviously the general state of health matters. The patient may be already rather frail, but in general the prognosis is not good.

Regular visiting of old people by relatives, by the good neighbour scheme, or by the reporting of any unusual happening may prevent a number of susceptible individuals becoming victims of hypothermia.

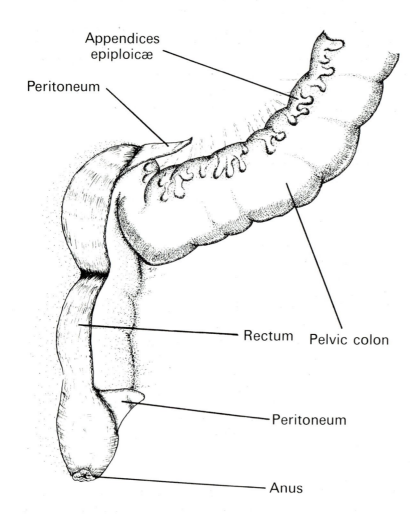

Appendices
epiploicæ

Peritoneum

Rectum   Pelvic colon

Peritoneum

Anus

31 Constipation

Constipation really means that there is some delay in the passage of faecal material through the large intestine, the chronic form being by far the most common, acute constipation usually being associated with intestinal obstruction.

The chronic type of constipation implies that there is some delay throughout the whole of the colon, or the delay occurs in the rectum. When the cause is due to lack of propulsive movements in the colon, or perhaps due to some mechanical defect, the type may be classed as chronic constipation. The term *dyschezia* is used when the delay occurs in the rectum.

Causes of colonic constipation

1 Lack of bulk in the diet either from lack of roughage in the diet or from insufficient intake of food resulting in poor peristalsis.
2 A colon which too readily absorbs water resulting in hard faeces.
3 Severe dehydration.
4 Hypertonic state of the muscles of the colon – spastic constipation.
5 Stricture of the bowel due to carcinoma.
6 Diverticulitis.

It must be remembered that individuals differ in the frequency in which their bowels are evacuated. Many have a bowel movement once or twice a day while others may feel no discomfort if an interval of two or three days elapses between bowel evacuations. Both routines would be compatible with normal health, consequently it is difficult to be precise in what constitutes constipation. Changes in bowel habits can be of significance, such changes occurring in carcinoma of the bowel when the increasing constipation will sometimes alternate with bouts of diarrhoea.

Dyschezia

Dyschezia is due to functional sluggishness of the bowel and can exist in individuals who persistently fail to answer the call to defaecate, resulting in large masses of faeces becoming impacted in the rectum. It frequently occurs in old people who may have some weakness of the muscles of the abdomen and pelvic floor thus creating lack of expulsive force. Other contributory factors may be due to improper toilet training in childhood, poor housing conditions where there is an insufficiency of lavatory accommodation, and also in patients who are confined to bed with a fractured femur, or other treatment which will necessitate their position in bed in the supine, or semi-recumbent position for relatively long periods. Nurses are well aware of the difficulties some patients experience with bedpans.

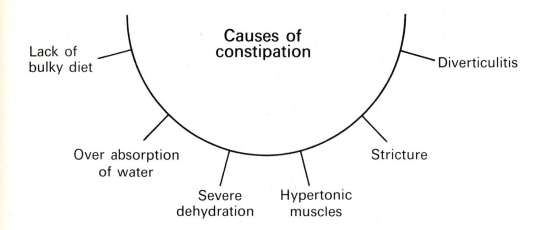

Causes of constipation

Lack of bulky diet

Over absorption of water

Severe dehydration

Hypertonic muscles

Stricture

Diverticulitis

Treatment

Re-educate the patient

Manual evacuation

Enemata

Laxatives

Purgatives

Treatment

When relevant the patient should be re-educated particularly when the cause is failure to answer the call to stool. It must be emphasised that attending the call will play its part in re-educating the bowel.

Some patients will have their own particular favourite pill or laxative and most doctors will allow them to continue their use whilst in hospital.

Perhaps the more difficult cases are the weak and elderly patients some of whom may require a manual evacuation of the rectum, followed by an enema later and probably the use of laxatives. Diet is obviously of importance, a diet with an increased amount of roughage will be of benefit i.e. one with sufficient green vegetables, fruit, and wholemeal bread.

Drugs

There are many drugs available for the relief of constipation but the condition is best treated whenever possible by modifying the diet.

Purgatives such as magnesium and sodium sulphate are useful on occasions for individuals who are not chronically constipated, but some people regularly take a small dose daily.

Other common drugs include paraffin emulsion which acts by softening stools, Dulcolax (Bisacodyl) which can be given orally or as a suppository, or preparations containing rhubarb, cascara or senna.

Some preparations e.g. methylcellulose act as a bulk purgative but also assist in softening the stool.

The nurse should try to educate her patients against excessive use of any laxative or purgative.

Infectious fevers

   The invasion of the
body by a bacterium
or virus

Entry being

by droplet   or ingestion

Incubation period

The time between the invasion
of body tissue and the onset
of clinical symptoms

32 Infectious fevers

The term infectious fever is by custom usually restricted to conditions which are spread by direct contact, i.e. from patient to patient. The term infectious disease can obviously be applied to any illness which has been caused by invasion of the body by micro-organisms but here the diseases considered will be those which have been caused by a specific bacterium or virus, and which in many cases confers a lasting immunity after one attack.

Incubation period
Most nurses will recall the term and its definition i.e. the time which elapses between the invasion of body tissues by the micro-organism and the onset of the clinical symptoms. Listed below are the incubation period for the diseases which will be discussed.

Measles (morbilli)	10–14 days.
Whooping cough (Pertussis)	10–14 days.
Chicken Pox (Varicella)	14–21 days.
German Measles (Rubella)	14–21 days.
Mumps (Epidemic Parotitis)	14–28 days.

Routes of infection
The causative organism is spread either by droplet infection or is taken in contaminated food or drink.

Quarantine period
This is usually a few days longer than the incubation period.

Notifiable diseases
Some infectious diseases *have* to be notified to the public health authorities but others are only notifiable under special circumstances, i.e. when large numbers have been infected as in an epidemic.

General features of acute infectious fevers
At the end of the incubation period the infecting organism or its toxic products give rise to the general features of the disease.

1 Pyrexia.
   The degree of pyrexia will vary and range from being moderate (37.2–38.2 C.) to being, in some instances, hyperpyrexial (40.5 C.)
2 Feeling of general malaise.
3 Restlessness.
4 Headache.
5 Loss of appetite.
6 Hot dry skin, dry furred tongue.

General features of infectious fevers

➤ Pyrexia
   Varying from 37.2PC – 40.5PC

➤ Malaise
   A general feeling of discomfort

➤ Restlessness

➤ Headache

➤ Loss of appetite

➤ Hot dry skin
   Furred tongue

➤ Diminished urinary output

➤ Increase in pulse rate &
   respiratory rate

➤ Constipation

➤ Other features may include
   a rash

7 Diminished urinary output.

8 Constipation.

9 Pulse rate and respiratory rate are usually above normal.

10 In addition to the above, other features will appear such as a typical rash, the appearance of the latter often enabling the physician to make his diagnosis.

Nursing care

Isolation or barrier nursing will be required to prevent any spread of infection. The nurse will ensure that all the usual basic nursing needs of the patient are carried out. She will ensure that the patients skin and pressure areas are attended to, oral toilet carried out and the fluid intake and nutritional needs of the patient are adequate.

All efforts are made to ensure the patient does rest and have adequate sleep. Unless otherwise indicated, the patient is nursed in the upright position or in the position he feels is most comfortable.

The room or cubicle will be well ventilated and free from draughts, the patients bed attire being chosen to ensure that when required for examination purposes it is easily removed.

Fluid charts and other nursing records are accurately kept, certain infectious diseases presenting a typical pattern of pyrexia. As the patient will not feel like eating in the early stages the fluid chart will show that adequate hydration is being maintained.

Measles

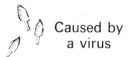 Caused by
a virus

By droplet
infection

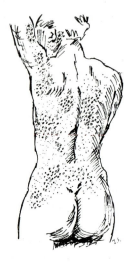

More commonly
a disease of
childhood

Incubation period
10 − 14 days

Clinical features

Early

Nasal catarrh
Photophobia & watery eyes
Conjunctivitis
Sneezing
Cough
Fever
Koplick's spots

After 3 − 4 days

Rash − First behind ears & forehead
then remainder of face & body

33 Measles (Morbilli)

Measles, a virus infection, is a common disease of childhood and next to whooping cough is perhaps the most serious infectious fever of early life.

A mother who has had measles will confer a passive immunity to her baby for the first three months of its life. Spread is by droplet infection, the condition being most prevalent in the first six months of the year, the incidence reaching its peak about March when widespread epidemics may occur.

The incubation period is 10–14 days following which the patient develops the symptoms of what appears to be a common cold.

The onset is sudden with the following symptoms being well in evidence.

1 Nasal catarrh.
2 Photophobia with watering of the eyes.
3 Conjunctivitis.
4 Sneezing.
5 Cough.
6 Fever.

Some patients may also develop laryngitis when hoarseness of the voice is present. During this time the diagnostic feature of measles can be seen inside the mouth, i.e. Koplik's spots. It is during this period that the disease is highly infectious. Three or four days later the Koplik's spots disappear and the dark red rash of the condition begins.

The temperature usually rises to 37.8°C–39.4°C on the first day, falls slightly on the second and rises again on the fourth with the appearance of the rash.

The rash has the particular feature of appearing first on the forehead and behind the ears but gradually spreads over the face and body, fading in about one week, the temperature also slowly falling over this period.

Treatment

Isolation in a well ventilated room is required, the position of the bed being away from the light because of the photophobia. Similarly, care of the eyes is necessary due to the conjuctivitis, any discharges being gently wiped away with warm saline. Oral toilet as a routine is also performed. Careful note of the respiratory rate will be made, any increase being reported as this may indicate the onset of one complication of the condition, i.e. bronchopneumonia. Penicillin or other antibiotics will be ordered to combat the infection. Should the child complain of pain in the ear, or the nurse notice any discharge this may be the result of secondary bacterial infection of the middle ear (otitis

Treatment

Isolation away from direct light

Care of the eyes

Antibiotics if prescribed

Care of the skin, bathing & calamine lotion

Observe respirations & ear pain for complications

Adequate fluids followed by a light diet

Complications

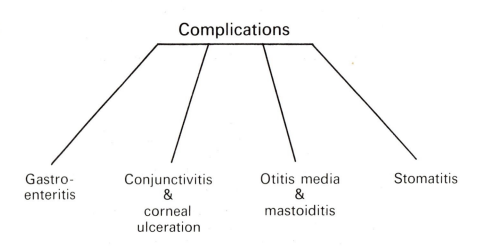

Gastro-enteritis

Conjunctivitis & corneal ulceration

Otitis media & mastoiditis

Stomatitis

media) and again antibiotics will be ordered. Severe inflammatory infections may require myringotomy which facilitates drainage.

Attention to the skin in the form of daily bed baths together with the application of a soothing lotion such as calamine to the rash will assist in making the patient more comfortable. The child is usually in bed for a few days but providing the room has an even temperature may get up when he feels like it. Milder cases may not require to be confined to bed for such a period.

The usual routine terminal disinfection for infectious disease is carried out.

Diet
Adequate fluid intake will be ensured in the early stages but later a light diet containing such foods as egg custards, fish, mince and scrambled eggs plus extra milk will be given.

Complications
Bronchopneumonia which as indicated above is the most serious complication particularly in the very young. Other complications include:
1 Gastro enteritis.
2 Conjunctivitis with corneal ulceration.
3 Otitis media leading to mastoiditis.
4 Stomatitis.
More rarely encephalitis which is inflammation of the brain and encephalomyelitis which means inflammation of the brain and spinal cord.

Immunisation
Passive immunity to measles can be achieved by giving an injection of gamma globulin a preparation which contains the antibodies to measles. This could be given to contacts, and if given within five days of exposure will prevent the onset of the condition. This immunity will last for about three weeks.

Active immunity. Measles vaccines are now available whereby an injection of live attenuated measles virus is given to children over one year of age who have not had the disease.

Rubella

More common in adolescents &
young adults

Incubation — 18 days

Small pink macular
rash on forehead
and behind
the ears

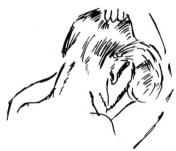
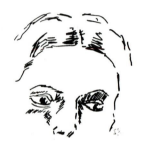

Enlargement of
lymph nodes &
joint tenderness

Point to note for females

Infection during the early months of
pregnancy can affect the foetus

Immunisation is important between
the ages of 11 — 14 years

34 German measles (Rubella)

German measles is less infectious and spreads less readily than measles, the age group being somewhat different in that it affects older children, adolescents and young adults. It causes little constitutional upset but is of significance when acquired by women in the first four months of pregnancy when it may lead to developmental defects in the foetus. Such abnormalities as cardiac defects, mental defects, deafness or cateracts may result. All female nurses who have not had rubella are immunised prior to taking up training. It is also recommended that all girls who have not had rubella should be similarly vaccinated between the age of eleven and fourteen years. The cause is a virus spread by droplet infection.

Clinical features

The incubation period is usually about 18 days but sometimes the constitutional symptoms are so slight that the first indication of the disease is the rash. The spots are small pink macules which first appear on the forehead and behind the ears. These spots remain distinct and do not run together as seen in morbilli.

The other notable features of the condition are enlargement of the lymph nodes particularly the cervical group, and possibly some tenderness in the joints, a degree of fever is seen in certain cases. The rash disappears in about two to three days. There is no treatment of note, its main significance being the effects which may arise in early pregnancy.

Whooping cough

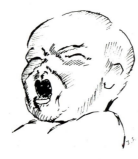

Caused by a bacterium

By droplet infection

Children under
5 years of age

Incubation period
7 – 14 days

Clinical features

A cold which develops into upper respiratory
tract infection

Paroxysms of coughing develop causing the
child to hold its breath

Followed by a long inspiration with the
resulting "whoop"

Complications

Acute bronchitis   Lobar pneumonia

Bronchiectasis   Convulsions

Otitis media

35 Whooping cough (Pertussis)

This highly infectious disease of the respiratory tract is caused by Bordetella pertussis and is spread by droplet infection. The disease is notifiable, and is still, perhaps, the most serious of the acute specific fevers of childhood, but the incidence and severity of the condition has been decreasing due to the prophylactic measures which can be taken.

Whooping cough occurs at all ages but the majority of cases are children under five years of age. Young infants receive no passive immunity from their mother and are consequently susceptible from birth. The incubation period is seven to fourteen days.

Clinical features

At first it appears as if the child has an ordinary cold which is actually a highly infective upper respiratory catarrh. This lasts for about one week in which rhinitis, conjunctivitis and an unproductive cough are in evidence. After a week the paroxysms of coughing are distinctive and there is no mistaking the nature of the disease. The child during the paroxysm is 'blue in the face', holds his breath for a while, then takes a long deep inspiration and the resulting 'whoop'. Vomiting may now occur and the child expectorates a thick, sticky mucus. A series of such bouts can occur and can number 30–40 in 24 hours, but they are much more severe at night time.

During very severe attacks the tongue can protrude to such an extent that the tongue can be abraded on the lower teeth and cause ulceration of the frenum.

The course of the disease usually lasts about three weeks with the bouts becoming less severe. The cough becomes less frequent and the sputum less tenacious. Following the disease there is usually lasting immunity.

Complications

Acute bronchitis and lobar pneumonia are the most serious complications. Plugs of mucus which block the bronchioles can cause bronchiectasis. Convulsions when they occur are of serious significance. A further complication which can arise is otitis media.

Treatment

The drug of choice is Tetracycline which can be given as a suspension to the child. Feeding and the maintenance of nutrition may present a problem but feeds may be retained if given immediately after the vomiting which the paroxysm of coughing causes. Some infants may require to be nursed in an oxygen tent. Phenobarbitone may also be ordered which may reduce the number of paroxysms and will have a calming effect.

Mumps

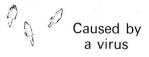 Caused by
a virus

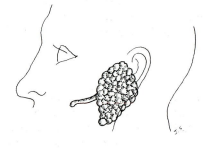 By droplet
infection

School children
& young
adults

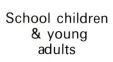

Incubation period
18 – 21 days

Clinical features

Fever

Swelling of parotid glands

Malaise

Complications

Orchitis
Oopheritis
Mastitis
Prostatitis
Meningitis

Isolation is
necessary until
glands are no
longer swollen

36 Mumps (Epidemic parotitis)

Mumps is caused by a virus and is spread by droplet infection, the age group being children of school age and young adults. The condition is relatively trivial but it can present serious complications if contracted after puberty. Most cases appear to occur in the spring and the incubation period is 18–21 days.

Clinical features
Fever.
Malaise.
Swelling of the parotid glands, which are tender.
The tender swelling of the salivary glands usually subsides after a few days, the temperature also reaches normal during this period.

Complications
Orchitis which is usually confined to one testicle is probably the most common complication. The patient complains of severe pain on the affected side and the teste is swollen and tender. Oophoritis results in the patient complaining of severe lower abdominal pain often accompanied by vomiting.

Other complications which may arise include mastitis, prostatitis and meningitis. The nurse will report any abdominal pain or if there are clinical signs of meningitis such as headache, vomiting, neck rigidity or drowsiness.

Treatment
No specific treatment is required but oral toilet is important. Feeding may be difficult if the patient cannot open the mouth but fluids can be given by means of a straw.

Should orchitis be present the physician will order some form of steroid drug which will give relief. The patient is isolated until all the glandular swelling has disappeared.

Chicken pox

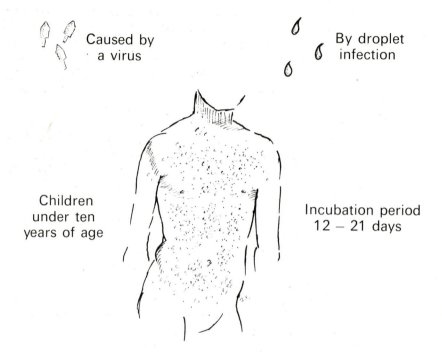

Caused by
a virus

By droplet
infection

Children
under ten
years of age

Incubation period
12 – 21 days

Clinical features

Rash appears on the trunk on the
second day.

A red papular rash which changes to
vesicles & pustules, followed by scabs.

The spots appear in crops and papules,
vesicles, pustules & scabs can appear at
the same time

37 Chicken pox (Varicella)

Chicken pox is nearly always a mild disease, the cause being a virus. The virus which causes chicken pox in children is closely allied to the virus which causes shingles in adults, or may be due to a reactivation of a latent infection. The incubation period is about 12–21 days but more usually around 14 days. A relatively common infection, the disease is more prevalent in autumn and winter. The condition is highly infectious, the most likely age group being children under ten years of age.

Clinical features
The child does not appear to be particularly unwell and the first sign of the disease may be the appearance of the rash. The particular features of the rash in chicken pox are as follows.
1 Appears on the trunk on the second day of the illness.
2 The red, papular rash quickly changes to vesicles and pustules which dry up after a few days causing scabs which quickly fall off.
3 The spots appear in crops, the nurse will observe that papules, vesicles, pustules and crusts will be seen in any area at the same time.

Initially the child will have a mild pyrexia and with vague feelings of malaise and a headache, the constitutional symptoms being therefore rather brief and mild.

Infection may ensue due to the patient scratching.

The physician will examine the patient carefully in order to exclude the more serious condition of smallpox. The condition can also be mistaken for a variety of skin diseases e.g. impetigo, scabies.

Treatment
Treatment is usually symptomatic. Skin irritations can be relieved by calamine lotion, the main concern being the prevention of any secondary infections.

The patient will be isolated until all the crusts have separated. Although mild in children, the disease can be more severe in adults.

Immunity

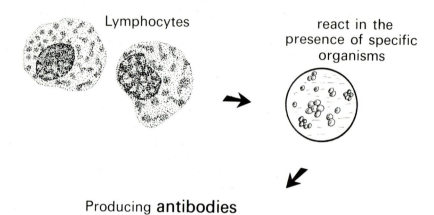

Lymphocytes

react in the
presence of specific
organisms

Producing **antibodies**
the antibody – antigen reaction

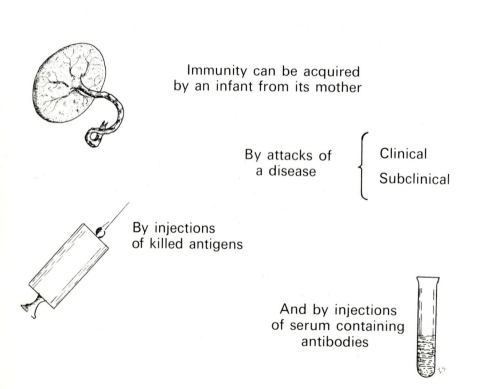

Immunity can be acquired
by an infant from its mother

By attacks of
a disease

{ Clinical

Subclinical

By injections
of killed antigens

And by injections
of serum containing
antibodies

38 Immunity

The body possesses its own protective mechanisms against the invasion of bacteria and other foreign agents. The protection given is either completely or partly successful in overcoming infections. Polymorphonuclear leucocytes for example which attack and ingest bacteria indiscriminately, will probably overcome micro-organisms but will not confer any lasting immunity.

The lymphocyte in lymphoid tissue and other special cells found in the plasma react somewhat differently in that they liberate chemical substances which have a *specific* effect on *specific* micro-organisms i.e. they produce antibodies to one particular disease. The causative agent whether bacteria or other foreign substances which cause the body to produce the antibodies or antitoxins is called an antigen. The response of the cells of the infected individual to the antigen and the production of antibodies is known as the Antibody — Antigen reaction. Three types of immunity are recognised.

1 Natural immunity. 2 Active immunity. 3 Passive immunity.

1 Natural acquired immunity
Resistance to disease may be inherited by antibodies from the mother passing to the infant. This form of immunity lasts only for a short time. Humans possess a natural immunity to some diseases of animals and vice versa.

2 Active immunity
This can be gained by:
I Suffering from a clinical attack of a disease and on recovery having naturally produced the specific antibodies to the disease OR
II Repeated subclinical attacks which do not produce all the characteristics of the disease but nevertheless have a sufficient antigen activity to produce antibodies resulting in active immunity.

Injection of the antigen which has been killed by heat or chemical means will, because the toxin has not been destroyed, stimulate the production of antibodies producing *artificially acquired* active immunity.

3 Passive immunity
Injections of serum containing the antibodies already present will confer passive immunity because the recipient has not actively produced the antibodies. Such immunity may be given to prevent infection in an individual exposed to the disease.
Diseases in which *artificial acquired immunity* is of value.
1 Diphtheria. 2 Tetanus. 3 Whooping cough. 4 Typhoid fever.
5 Poliomyelitis. 6 Tuberculosis. 7 Smallpox.
Diseases in which *passive immunity* is of value.
1 Diphtheria.   2 Measles.   3 Smallpox.

Prophylaxis

Active immunisation against whooping cough is available and is usually in the combined triple vaccine, i.e. whooping cough, diphtheria and tetanus. Very young infants are particularly susceptible consequently care is exercised in preventing these babies from any possible exposure.

Index